Staying Off the Diet Rollercoaster

Staying Off the Diet Rollercoaster

Linda Omichinski, R.D.

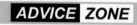

Washington, D.C.

AdviceZone books and audio-tapes may be purchased directly either from the AdvizeZone website at www.advicezone.com by calling toll-free at 1-800-210-ZONE.

Library of Congress Cataloging-in-Publication Data Omichinski, Linda, 1955–

Staying off the diet rollercoaster / Linda Omichinski p. cm.

Includes biographical references and index.

ISBN 0-9668725-4-1 (pbk: alk. paper)

1. Nutrition. 2. Diet. 3. Self-care, Health. 4. Physical Fitness. 5. Reducing-Safety measures. 6. Reducing diets. I. Title.

RA784 .O545 2000

613.7-dc21

This book is intended as an educational and informational resource. The publisher and author expressly disclaim any responsibility or liability in connection with the use of this book.

Cover design by Bookwrights.com, Charlottesville, VA, Mayapriya Long. Interior design by Nancy Gratton and by Publishing Professionals, New Port Richey, FL, Sylvia Hemmerly.

Cover photograph by Allan Montaine/Photonica

DEDICATION

To my dear parents, whose "I love you" hugs, "I'm so proud of you" smiles, and "I believe in you" looks of reassurance have given me the confidence to be who I am today. To my mother-in-law, who gave me the encouragement to be all that I could be. To my husband Mitchell, may your dreams come true as you have allowed mine to come true. And to the dieters of the world, that you find the guidance and freedom you need to transfer your newfound energy into a meaningful way of living.

ACKNOWLEDGMENTS

This book has brought many special people's insights, talents, and expertise into play. My deepest thanks goes out to all of them: To Sandra Barsy, whose six years of dedication to the *HUGS Club News*, the inspiration for this book, made taking this next step possible. Thank you Sandra for hanging in there, for the input, guidance, and direction that you have provided along the way. To Heather Wiebe Hildebrand, Penny Muir, Christie Keating, Becky Chase, Sandra Olafson, and Kerri Miller, all of whom add their expertise to the pages of this book. Thanks also to Linda Bacon and Joanne Ikeda, for checking on the accuracy of some sections of the book, and to Joanne particularly for her review of the book as a whole. Also thanks to Alice Ansfield of *Radiance Magazine* for her contribution to the book and for reviewing the finished manuscript, and thanks to Francie Berg for writing the Foreword and for her many years of support. A huge thank-you to many other contributors of the book: Heidi Mead, Shelley McDonald, Tanis Rempel, Heather Todd, Carol Johnson, Linda Mayoh, and Wendyl Niessen. And a special thanks to Sandra Storen, whose cartoon illustrations took my written words and made them work artistically. Thanks to Janis Jibrin and Nancy Gratton, who together helped edit the manuscript, and to my publishing team, Michelle Tullier and especially Nathanial Jackson of AdviceZone. Last but not least, thanks to the long-term supporters of my work: my parents, Catherine and Steve Thoman; my husband Mitchell; and my mother-in-law Vicki Omichinski, thank you for being there. I'd like to also acknowledge those special people in my life who have helped in numerous ways: Valerie Giesbrecht, Karen Graham, Jan Rempel, and many others too numerous to mention. Your contribution is well appreciated.

TABLE OF CONTENTS

Foreword	viii
Preface	x
Welcome to Your New Life	1
Remembering Why You Stopped Dieting	13
Ditching the Diet Dialog	31
Lose Weight and Call Me in the Morning	47
Support Yourself	59
Resetting Your Stress Barometer	71
A Self-Esteem Shot in the Arm	89
Getting Back into Exercise	111
Making Exercise a Lifelong Affair	127
Tuning into Hunger and Thirst	139
The Guided Journal	155
Tailoring Your Tastes	175
Next Stop: Buddy Support	199
Appendix A	217
Appendix B	221
Index	223
Bibliography	225

FOREWORD

Riding the diet rollercoaster—on again, off again, losing weight and regaining it—is no way to go through life. It's time to get off, to start life anew as a healthier, happier person. *Staying off the Diet RollerCoaster* shows the way. This book urges us to nurture and nourish ourselves, to trust our bodies, to eat and live actively for health, not for thinness, and to enjoy health and well-being at the size we are. The author, Linda Omichinski, is a pioneer in the nondiet, size-accepting, health-at-any-size movement. For more than a decade she has brought her positive message of pleasurable, diet-free living to people around the world. It's a revolutionary message for our times. The thinness obsession that grips our culture today, puts enormous pressure on women, and increasingly on men, to reduce and reshape their bodies.

The media's "ideal woman" has shrunk by nearly a third in the past 30 years, as revealed in studies of how Miss America contestants and Playboy centerfolds have become painfully thinner, year by year. In response, many women are making their bodies their life's work. More are eating in disordered, dysfunctional ways. Statistics show that, at any given time, over half of women and girls, and a quarter of men and boys, are trying to lose weight by dieting, skipping meals, fasting, bingeing, or exercising obsessively. Even children are using dangerous methods—vomiting, taking laxatives, diuretics, diet pills, or smoking. One-fourth of teenage girls are severely undernourished. Eating disorders are increasing, and striking at ever younger ages.

All this comes at a stiff price—in weakness, fatigue, inability to focus or function well, irregular heart beat, and sometimes death. Meanwhile, the incidence of obesity is also increasing. There is evidence that dieting, weight cycling, and the disruption of normal eating often lead to excess weight gain. Size prejudice, too, is on the upswing, and it serves to keep people committed to dieting. The good news is that there is a better way. In this book and through her organization, HUGS International, Linda brings a clear message of healthy eating, active living, self-acceptance, and an appreciation of diversity in others. She empowers people, assuring us all that we each have the solution within ourselves, if we will but nourish it. Learning to eat when hungry and stop when full offers a life of freedom, an opportunity to rediscover and use our body-wisdom.

Linda's voice is consistent, caring, reassuring, and informed. She is confident that the diet-free approach is the better way. Her confidence is firmly based upon an intimate knowledge of the dieting model. During her early years as a dietitian, she practiced traditional diet counseling, helping patients lose weight through programs that restricted food. When they gained it back, she shared their frustration and, unlike other health providers who continued to use failed approaches, she soon began to look for a better way. She found it by moving away from diets. She developed the HUGS program, now facilitated by dietitians and other health professionals in Canada, the United States, and several other countries. Through her books, programs, and online activities, Linda reaches out to people around the globe, empowering them to discover safer, saner, healthier ways to think about their bodies and their weight.

This book teaches readers how to rid themselves of the diet mentality, tune in to hunger and thirst, tailor their tastes to enjoy nutritious foods, build self-esteem, and manage stress. It explains the importance of physical activity and the joys of journaling. It offers advice on working with (and converting) health providers and strengthening support networks. The real life experiences shared throughout the book help bring Linda's concepts to life. Personal stories bring us the voices of women struggling to maintain healthy lifestyles despite difficulties, providing gentle words of empathy and encouragement for those times when staying off the diet rollercoaster gets hard. A pleasurable read, this is also a self-help book that anyone can use, whether working alone or in a group.

Staying Off the Diet Rollercoaster reminds us that fitness is within everyone's grasp—and it doesn't take a lifetime membership in the local gym to achieve it. Instead, it tells us that healthy eating, moderate but regular activity, and a strong personal support network can help everyone find a fulfilling, diet-free lifestyle. It has been said that one person can make a difference; two or three working together can make a miracle. Linda Omichinski not only makes a difference in people's lives; she has marshaled a network of visionary health care providers working together to bring forth that miracle. We can be assured this book will extend and strengthen that network. The world is a better place because of Linda's dedication and passion to the cause of better living for everyone.

Francie M. Berg, MS, Editor, *Healthy Weight Journal*, Adjunct Professor, University of North Dakota School of Medicine

PREFACE

What's this? A dietitian who won't put you on a diet? That's me! But I wasn't always such a revolutionary. Back when I was first starting out, I did what all registered dietitians were taught to do: I equated losing weight with improving health, and prescribed—you guessed it—diets to many of my clients. Until, one day, I had an amazing revelation. For awhile I had listened uncritically to my clients as they told me how happy they were with the individualized diets I designed for them. "I never feel deprived" they would claim. Or they'd tell me: "I'm really losing weight on this plan." But then, one day, it hit me: sooner or later I'd lose contact with them for awhile, only to run into them in the local grocery store—where they were invariably embarrassed because they'd gained the weight back.

After a few such encounters I realized the simple truth—dieting *just doesn't work*! What was I to do? My training obviously had ignored something very important—so I set out to discover what that "something" was. I hit the books, of course, but I also started listening—*really* listening—to my clients. And that's how I came to my first breakthrough: I realized that the only way to achieve lasting weight-loss results was to *stop* all this obsessive focusing on diets! A revolutionary concept! Losing weight by NOT dieting!

For lots of people, it was also a concept that seemed to contradict how they expected things to work in the real world. But if you think about it, this idea—like all great ideas—is based on some simple truths. Diets don't work because they make you feel bad about yourself. They almost *force* you to obsess about the very thing that causes you problems—food! And they set you up for a series of failures: starving, starving, starving until you drop a few pounds; then you can't take the deprivation anymore, so you binge, binge, binge until all the weight comes right back—usually with a few (or more than a few) extra!

So I became part of a new, non-diet movement. My new approach did away with dieting altogether, and focused instead on making positive lifestyle changes. I felt that as my clients developed more positive self-images, and learned healthy food and exercise habits, weight loss would naturally follow. In 1987, arising directly out of this new movement, came HUGS. At first it was a single class and information center in my hometown of Portage la Prairie, Manitoba, Canada. While my early rejection of dieting was a big break from the traditional nutrition establishment, however, it was only a first step. After all, I still was focusing on the goal of weight loss. But I was also still listening to my clients—and I was slowly beginning to believe that there was something missing in my approach. One client finally put the whole problem into perspective. She said to me: "Linda, I'm no longer starving and bingeing. I'm eating more regularly. I'm beginning to actually prefer healthier foods, and I feel the increased energy those foods bring to me. I'm even enjoying walking for the fun of it. But *I am not losing weight*! What am I doing wrong?"

The woman asking me this question stood in front of me, fairly *glowing* with good health, looking strong and fit—and she thought that she had failed! That's when it hit me—when I realized what had been missing in the program up to that point. I said: "You're not doing *anything* wrong. You may simply be at the weight your body was meant to be." And the full philosophy behind today's HUGS International was born! You see—in this culture, we're trained to think that we have to be thin to be healthy, happy, attractive, and worthwhile. We're trained to believe that our success and value are determined by the number that shows up when we stand on the bathroom scale. But that training is wrong! We all have different body shapes, metabolisms, and activity levels. People are *not* meant to be "one size for all." And with that realization, I knew what it would take to make HUGS not just revolutionary, but truly inspirational. Just as I did away with diets, I now proposed to do away with the focus on weight loss entirely.

You see, the old, traditional diet mentality has everything backwards. It places the focus on weight loss and makes getting healthier a kind of bonus prize. The HUGS program, on the other hand, turns that philosophy upside down: getting healthier is our focus, and weight loss is the bonus that often comes when you adopt a healthier lifestyle. I brought this new, matured philosophy to my HUGS classes, and the next thing you know, class participants began asking if I had a book, video, or other support materials they could buy. In 1992 I published *You Count, Calories Don't*, and the momentum for my non-diet program really took off!

Today, my little local program of classes has grown—it's now called HUGS International, Inc., to reflect the fact that we have a network of groups spread across Canada, the U.S., New Zealand, South Africa, and the U.K.! We ran into some opposition from the nutrition establishment at the outset, but that was only to be expected, given how entrenched the diet mentality is in our culture and society. Just like my clients, the establishment itself needed to be educated to this new approach—so I published articles in professional journals and brought the HUGS message to professional nutritionist and dietitian conferences. Over time, the value of the HUGS non-diet program gained the professional respect it deserved.

At HUGS, we teach people how to live a balanced, healthy lifestyle, in which they learn to feel good about themselves no matter what the bathroom scales say. In fact, that's how the program got its name—after all, the universal response to a hug is to feel good, loved, worthwhile. Lots of people ask just what the letters stand for, and some have tried to guess—my favorite is the woman who was *sure* it stood for "Human Understanding through Group Support." But I'll let you in on a little secret—it doesn't stand for *anything*—it's just a great big HUG, with capital letters to show how big a HUG you can learn to give yourself, once you've been through the program.

So, you may be asking, just what *is* this magical program? In terms of its nuts-and-bolts, it's a series of 10 group counseling sessions, led by a licensed professional and based on the principles laid down in my book, *You Count, Calories Don't*. These sessions are backed up by a post-program support system that uses this book. This volume, and the HUGS Web site (look for HUGS at www.hugs.com) are also an important part of the program. Each year, HUGS reaches out to thousands of participants, who come to us to learn how to begin a diet-free lifestyle. So, whether you're reading this book as a curious newcomer interested in learning the HUGS philosophy, a current HUGS participant, or a HUGS veteran looking for some post-program support, welcome! This book is written for all of you—to bring you into the warm embrace of a healthier, happier, way of life!

Linda Omichinski

Welcome to Your New Life 1

Time to Make a Change
Where Are You Right Now?
    The diet mentality quiz
    Scoring yourself
    Get ready for a change
    Gauging your state of change
A Philosophy of Change
Real Life Measures of Success
Taking It Deeper

I have a simple goal: I want to change your life! I want to help make you a happier, healthier person. I'm hoping to show you how to achieve the most beautiful makeover you've ever had.

How are you going to achieve this makeover? By shucking the oppressive diet mentality and starting life all over again—this time as a saner, healthier, happier person. Some of you have already left that old calorie-counting mentality behind. If so, this book will provide the reinforcement you need to keep from going back there. I hope to convince you that the diet rollercoaster—dieting, going off the diet, feeling guilty and worthless, going back on the diet—is no way to go through life. But whether you're already off that rollercoaster or still trying to dismount, you need support. That's what this book is all about.

Time to Make a Change?

Have you stopped exercising? Found yourself eating a lot more sweets? Starting to think that Jenny Craig may be the only solution? I know how tough it is to fend off the urge to diet in the face of the constant pressure from the multi-billion-dollar weight-loss and advertising industries. Not to mention the demands of your busy life, which make it hard to find the time to exercise and eat right. But before you give up, try this book first. You don't have to read it all; simply turn to the chapters that meet your immediate needs to help you get back in balance. Then come back later to see what else I've got to offer. Your goal, and mine: to discover a healthy lifestyle without ever dieting again.

If you're new to a lifestyle without diets, don't panic. You may be thinking: "Does this mean I'll *never* lose weight?" Not at all. The nondiet approach emphasizes

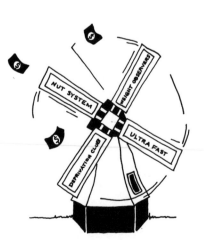

health instead of weight, but as you adopt a healthier lifestyle, you probably will lose your extra pounds. But even if you don't, you'll learn how to allow yourself to enjoy life instead of putting it on hold until after you've lost the weight.

There's one thing I want to stress right from the start. As you'll notice as soon as you delve into this book, I've abandoned the usual measures of "dieting success." You'll find no scales, no tape measure, no questions about how loose your jeans are.

These are all no-win standards of measuring success, because every dieter fails them, time and time again. Instead, I focus on your attitudes as markers of progress: your attitude toward your body, toward food, toward your self-worth, toward your joy in living.

That said, are you ready to get started?

Where Are You Right Now?

You're about to discover two things about yourself: how entrenched you are in the diet mentality, and how ready you are to change. To help you address the first issue, I'm starting you out with a "Diet Mentality" quiz. This quiz has been scientifically validated as an accurate reading of how steeped you are in the diet mentality.

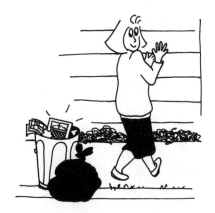

Take this quiz to get a snapshot of where you are now. But don't stop there! In Appendix B you'll find more blank copies of the quiz. Do a re-take after you've finished reading a few chapters, and take it once again when you're done with the entire book. Other good times to retake the quiz would be when you join a nondiet support group or when you link up with a nondieting buddy. That way you'll have a way to compare your before and after snapshots and see how you've progressed.

The diet mentality quiz

Score: 1 = always; 2 = very often; 3 = often; 4 = sometimes; 5 = rarely; 6 = never

_____ I am unhappy with myself the way I am.

_____ I am preoccupied with a desire to be thinner.

_____ I weigh myself several times a week.

_____ I am more concerned with the number on the scale than my overall sense of well-being.

_____ I think about burning up calories when I exercise.

The diet mentality quiz, cont'd	

_____ I am out of tune with my body for natural signals of hunger and fullness.

_____ I eat for other reasons than physical hunger.

_____ I eat too quickly, not taking time to focus on my meal and taste, savor and enjoy my food.

_____ I fail to take time for activities for myself.

_____ I fluctuate between periods of sensible, nutritious eating and out-of-control eating.

_____ I give too much time and thought to food.

_____ I tend to skip meals, especially early in the day, so I can "save up" my food for one big feast.

_____ I engage in all-or-nothing thinking.

_____ I try to be all things to all people.

_____ I strive for perfection in my life.

_____ I criticize myself for not achieving my goals.

Scoring yourself

Add up all the numbers. Add 4 to your total. The result is your Diet Mentality score. Here's what it means:

Between 0 and 24: You are entrenched in the diet mentality. Since most of society is in the same boat, don't feel bad. Congratulations for taking the first step to leave that diet thinking behind. This book will help you break free. Just remember: Your life is in the balance!

Between 25 and 49: You are still a diet thinker, very preoccupied with food and with your weight. You let numbers—calorie counts and portion sizes—rule you. If you have been dieting all your life, it takes time to break the diet mentality. But if you work through this book one step at a time and retake the test periodically, you'll be able to watch your scores improve.

Between 50 and 74: Good for you! You're well on your way to living a lifestyle without diets! You've already seen a shift in your thinking, and as a result even your behavior is beginning to change—for the healthier! But even though you are becoming less preoccupied with food and weight, you still have areas you need to work on. Look carefully at those areas in which you entered low scores, turn to the chapters that focus on those issues, and make sure to take the time to work through the Taking It Deeper sections.

Between 75 and 100: Bravo! Congratulations on entering the wonderful, healthy world of nondieters. Sure, you still indulge a little diet thinking from time to time, but that's totally normal. You are definitely on the right road to better health, and you have a healthy attitude toward food, weight, and life.Where are you in the stages of change right now? Since you're reading this book, you're probably already at Stage 2—you're at least contemplating the possibility of making a change. Now's the time to assess how ready you are to move on to the next stage. Are you content to let yourself move along the stages naturally, or are you hoping to boost yourself ahead a bit?

Get ready for a change

Earlier I mentioned that this chapter will help you assess two things about your own diet mentality: Where do you stand right now? And how ready are you to make a change? The quiz you just took gave you the answer to the first question. Now here's a chart that will help you answer the second. The first column describes the classic stages of readiness for change adapted from the "Stages of Change" model developed by Brian P. Dutton.

What's important to remember is that real change takes lots of time, and it's sometimes hard to see. You might find it helpful to look at earlier stages and try to assign dates to when you passed through them. Remember, in the nondieting approach the old measures of success—the scales—are no longer valid. Instead, your focus is on developing an improved attitude and becoming more skilled in crisis management. But progress in these areas often goes unnoticed. By tracking your movement along the various stages of change, you can spotlight your improvements and reinforce your will to succeed.

Oh, and while we're on the subject of tracking your progress, note that the relapse stage is considered a normal part of the change process. This is actually very comforting to many people, because it means you don't have to feel like a failure if you temporarily go off course. What's important is that, when you hit the relapse phase, you take the time to look closely at what knocked you off track. Then simply move on to whichever phase will most likely help you get back on track. It's also important to look closely for signs of success that you may have missed or forgotten.

Gauging Your State of Change

Classic model of change	Applied to getting off the diet rollercoaster
Stage 1: Pre-contemplation—I'm not even thinking about changing my behavior or thinking.	Dieting.
Stage 2: Contemplation—I'm not doing anything differently but I'm seriously considering making some changes in the next six months.	Frustrated and aware that dieting doesn't work.
Stage 3: Preparation—I'm not doing anything different but I plan to in the next thirty days, and I've tried over the past year.	Find out about alternatives, educate yourself.
Stage 4: Action—I'm doing some things differently but this is new for me, only over the past six months.	Buy resources to help you get off the diet rollercoaster; perhaps take a program.
Stage 5: Maintenance—I've changed my behavior and have maintained that change for more than six months.	After the book, after the program, a lifestyle without diets won't work without support. Get support.
Relapse—I'm having trouble maintaining changes and feel I'm slipping into old patterns. Although discouraging, relapse is a normal aspect of change. Most people cycle through stages several times before experiencing maintenance.	It's spring. You went back on another diet. You're feeling discouraged—don't be! It's quite normal to go back to old patterns, especially when you are trying to make a change for the first time. Find out what motivated you to go back once more. Look again at why you decided to stop dieting and reclaim your nondiet attitude. Move to whichever phase will put you back on track.

A Philosophy of Change

Dieting is, for many people, an exercise in frustration—not to mention that it can seriously hurt your sense of self-esteem *AND* your health. That's why, back in 1987, I started my HUGS program. My goal was to help people discover a safer, saner, healthier way to think about their bodies and their weight. And over time, HUGS has reached out to thousands of people around the globe, helping them to succeed in finding a healthy lifestyle—without diets.

Like the HUGS program, this book is a balance of inspiration and advice. You will read "Herstories"—the stories of actual people—people like you—who will take you into the pages of their own lives. Each chapter focuses on a different challenge in your journey of maintaining a healthy lifestyle, and offers articles by people like yourself—people who are living a lifestyle without diets. Each chapter also offers a section at the end that I call "Taking It Deeper." Here you'll find questions and exercises that allow you to reflect upon the issues raised in the chapter. By working through these exercises, you can probe more deeply into the issues that affect your attitudes to your health, weight, and happiness.

Here's how to make this book work for you:

- Read the chapter material to increase your knowledge and understanding about developing a healthy lifestyle.

- Identify with the "Herstories"—I promise you'll find advice and observations that are relevant to your own situation.

- Work through the "Taking It Deeper" questions to stimulate your progress. One good way to do this is to use the questions to inspire keeping a journal (see Chapter 11) that records your growth. Since I've found that telling someone else increases your likelihood of creating a personal action plan, I suggest that you also use these questions to get a discussion going with friends who share your goals, or in the context of a formally organized support group.

While this book can provide you with a good jumping-off point in your quest to get off the dieting rollercoaster, don't stop here! There are many other excellent support tools at your disposal:

- Check out the various online support options available to you at hugs.com. There you'll find message board posts, chat room exchanges, and potential e-mail buddying—all designed to enable you to get what you need when you need it.

- Try audio affirmations, available through HUGS (check the back of this book for order forms for this and other HUGS materials). These are effective tools for change and they can work hand-in-hand with the advice given in this book. Among other benefits, they'll help you to reframe your negative attitudes by helping you develop positive self-talk. What's more, this skill can be invaluable when transferred to other areas of your life.

- Gather with others for a support group to grow your lifestyle. Discussion focused on the "Taking It Deeper" questions from each chapter will ensure that your group is engaged in enabling, rather than complaining.

- Read other books to support your new, nondieting lifestyle. *You Count, Calories Don't* was my first book, written to give you a deeper understanding of the nondieting concept, and it gives you lots of practical ideas to help you make the change. Another useful book, which I co-authored with Heather Wiebe Hildebrand, is *Tailoring Your Tastes*. This is the HUGS concept cookbook, which teaches you how to acquire a taste for foods that are lower in fat, sugar, and salt and higher in fiber. Once you've retrained your palate, you'll find that you are eating these kinds of selections by choice, not because "your diet made you do it."

Enjoy the journey.

Real Life Measures of Success, *by Penny Muir*

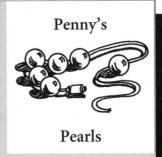

Penny's

Pearls

It's January again. Start of a new year, a new century, and a new millennium. Judging from various forms of media—newspaper, magazine, television, and radio—it would appear that not a lot has changed. There is a quiet stir of nondiet thinking beginning to surface, but it's still in its infancy.

Weight-loss advertisements are still everywhere. Fitness club parking lots are still packed with cars. My neighbors are still bundling up and braving the elements to get in a brisk daily walk. By mid February, however, this diet- and fitness-consciousness should begin to taper off and things will return to "normal."

The start of a new year is a good time to reflect and take stock of my life up to now, and it's a great time to look forward and set new goals. My 1997 New Year's resolution was to lose weight. My 1998 resolution was to put the HUGS philosophy into practice and to spread the word about the nondiet lifestyle. In 1999 I resolved to find a balance between being a Mom, a Wife, and a Woman. But this year, I didn't make a resolution at all. Instead, I spent some time taking stock of how I've changed over the past 3 years, and how I've learned to cope with real life situations.

I took my first "HUGS For Better Health" class in the spring of 1997. By January 1998 I had put some of the lessons into practice. I was seeing positive changes in my lifestyle and my attitude. But it hadn't translated very much into a visible change—I mean, I hadn't lost any weight or changed a dress size. And I was having trouble getting family and friends to listen to my ideas without seeing a glazed look come over their eyes. In fact, many times I thought HUGS wasn't working for me, because there weren't any real tangible results to measure my success by.

I stuck with it, though. I read and re-read *You Count, Calories Don't*, by HUGS founder Linda Omichinski, I don't know how many times. I pulled out my "HUGS at Home" tapes and listened to them countless times. With help from Linda, I got over some rough spots. In time, I took on some official HUGS functions and began to monitor the message board at the HUGS web site. I began providing e-mail mentoring for other HUGS graduates and participants. I took up the International No-Diet Day project and loved it. I was having a good time while learning and moving along my own HUGS journey.

One of the most important positive changes I've made is this: the scales no longer rule my mood. I still keep them in my powder room, however—they're digital, and I think they weigh accurately. But more often than not, they begin a discussion about HUGS with visitors to my home. It's funny how many of my friends and family go into that room and come out practically yelling at me about my "damn scales"—they seem to think it registers 4 pounds too heavy. I just laugh and say "Go ahead and believe that they weigh heavy, if that makes you feel better." But it *doesn't* make them feel better—instead, it often leads to a brief discussion about HUGS.

It's been a long journey, two years since I really started to work through HUGS and almost three years since I took the ten week program. In that time, I've learned that there are better indicators of my progress than the numbers on the scale. I've also learned that I sometimes still indulge in diet thinking—like looking for proof of my progress that others can easily see. But, most importantly, I've learned that every day is part of the process. Whether I have a "good" day or a "bad" one, I'm still learning and growing and moving along. I've hit some snags along the way, and sometimes I've moved in a direction that I thought was backwards. Many times over the three years I've even thought about going to a weight-loss program for a jumpstart. I've considered talking to my doctor about the latest in weight-loss drug treatments. I looked in the health-food stores at the herbal remedies for obesity and weight-loss treatments—but I always came back to HUGS.

I noticed how far I've really come the week between Christmas and New Year's. It was a difficult time—my father, from whom I'd been estranged for about the last four years, died on Christmas Day. Going to the funeral was going to be a family reunion of sorts—I hadn't seen many of my relatives since long before I was even married—when I was still thin. Before HUGS, this would have been a time of great insecurity for me—I'd have worried about what people thought of how I looked. But on the morning of the funeral I opened the closet, chose my clothes without a second thought, dressed, and left the house. I went through the process of the day and did what needed to be done.

It wasn't until I went to bed that night that I realized that I hadn't once thought about how I looked or how I would be perceived by people I hadn't seen in a long time. I hadn't had to struggle about what to wear, since I only have clothes that fit perfectly. I hadn't stewed about how big I had become. I hadn't felt ashamed of myself or my size. My attention and emotions were focused on the task at hand—and *not at all* on chastising or berating myself.

In spite of the emotional rollercoaster I'd been on during the days since my father's death, I fell asleep that night smiling and feeling happy with myself. Next morning, I took stock of how I'd handled my emotions over the past few days. I was happy to notice that my eating habits had not suffered: I hadn't tried to stuff down my feelings with food, nor had I lost my appetite because of bad nerves. Instead, my thoughts had been focused on the proper things—on grieving for my lost father, and on compassion for my siblings. I had faced everything head on.

I'm truly surprised by how far I've come in three years. Living a nondiet lifestyle has become so automatic that I have to force myself to sit back and take notice of the progress I've made. And, judging by the change in the number on the scale a week or two ago, even the visual results of my new way of life are beginning to show. I think that people around me are going to see what will look to them like a sudden change and maybe that will enable me to finally get them to listen to me when I talk about HUGS.

I'm not thrilled to realize that it will take a change in my body size for them to take me seriously, but then I have to acknowledge that this has been a very personal journey—one of self-discovery and self-gratitude. I've done the hard work and it's paid off for me in ways I never would have believed: It's changed my attitude; it's changed how I behave; it's changed how I treat myself and others; and it's changed how I react to things, both good and bad. There were times when I wanted to give it up and go back to the diet way. I'm so glad that I stuck with it and kept trudging along, even when it seemed impossible.

The longest, hardest part of the journey is now fully behind me and I'm looking forward to a new future. I don't mind looking back. It shows me how far I've come. When I turn around to look forward again the road ahead doesn't appear to be so long. I don't feel like I'm facing a goal that keeps moving away from me. I'm there. Now I have time to enjoy where I am.

Taking It Deeper

- **On: The Diet Mentality Quiz**

  1. Take a good look at your quiz responses. Which areas does it suggest that you need to work on most? Start thinking about how you might try to make some positive changes.

- **On: Your Stage of Change**

  1. By picking up this book, you've already shown that you are determined to stop dieting. The question now is just *how* ready you are. Review the various stages of change and consider how you might move along to greater readiness.

  2. The first step in problem solving is to clearly identify the problem and that's what you've just done. The next step is to think about how this model of change readiness can apply to other areas of your life.

- **On: Real Life Measures of Success**

  1. Plot Penny's movement through the various stages of the readiness-for-change model. Sometimes she slipped backward a bit—can you spot where this happens? Discuss how she has even managed to turn the backward movement into an opportunity for growth.

  2. Penny describes a three-year journey to get to a nondiet lifestyle where food and scales don't rule her. Discuss how her attitude has changed and how these changes have helped her deal with even difficult everyday situations positively. What parallels do you see between her experiences and the experiences of your own life?

Remembering Why You Stopped Dieting

2

The Ugly Side of Dieting
    Weight regain, and more
    Muscle loss
    The water-weight mirage
    A bane to beauty
    Bringing on bingeing
    Losing touch with your body's wisdom
    Misplaced priorities
    Hurts the heart and other vital organs
    Fertility problems
    Personality problems
    Skews your "set point"
So Let's Do Away with Dieting
Top Ten Reasons to Give Up Dieting
Making the Break
The Diet-Free Option
Ten Steps Toward Losing the Diet Mentality
The Label Trap
An International Perspective

W hat made you hop aboard the diet rollercoaster, last time around? Maybe it was the skinny woman your husband was talking to at the party last night. Or maybe it happened somewhere around page 50 of this month's *Vogue*—suddenly you were seized with "fat panic," and all you wanted to do was drop as many pounds as possible as soon as possible. "Fad diet, here I come!"

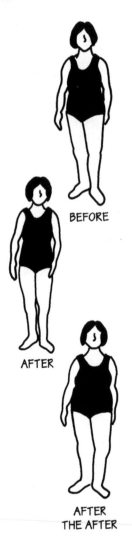

BEFORE

AFTER

AFTER
THE AFTER

It's easy to forget that diets don't work when you're seized with that kind of panic about your weight. But that's what this chapter is all about—to remind you why diets that promise quick weight loss aren't a good idea. So sit down, take a deep breath, and read this chapter carefully. When you're done, you'll understand that while there's nothing wrong with wanting to lose excess weight, there *is* something seriously wrong with dieting.

The Ugly Side of Dieting

For years, losing weight has meant dieting—too often, *fad* dieting. Even nutritionists sometimes fell into the trap of treating weight loss and health as synonymous. But all that has changed. Now health and nutrition professionals recognize that dieting has a dark side. And this knowledge has begun to make it out into the mainstream. For example, the California-based quarterly, *Radiance Magazine* (www.radiancemagazine.com)—which focuses on women's health and lifestyle issues—published a 1987 article that breaks down of some of the very real dangers of dieting. In this article, originally titled "Ten Reasons Not to Diet," author Ruth Priest listed the following health concerns:

Weight regain, and more

Ironically, dieting may not only leave you right back at your pre-diet weight. It might even make you heavier. Scientific studies document that 95 to 97 percent of persons who lose weight on the traditional diet route (calorie restrictive diets, with or without any increase in physical activity) gain the weight back within five years. My experience has been that when I ask an audience how many have been on diets and yet are heavier today than when they started dieting, most people raise their hands.

Muscle loss

When you drop your calorie intake low enough for the body to think it's starving, it draws sustenance from both fat and muscle. This means that you not only lose fat, you also lose some of your lean tissue. Losing lean muscle not only makes you weaker, it also lowers your metabolism. This, paradoxically, causes your body to burn fewer calories, making it easier to gain the weight right back. Even worse, when you gain back the weight, you run the risk of winding up with an even higher fat-to-muscle ratio than you had *before* you went on the diet!

The water-weight mirage

Don't be fooled—much of the weight you lose during the first few weeks of dieting is water weight, not fat. Here's how it works: When your calorie level drops too low, your body turns first to its carbohydrate stores in search of fuel—in this case, glycogen. Glycogen, however, is bound up with a lot of water—in fact, about three times its weight *is* water. So, as your body uses up its glycogen, you can also lose 3, 5, 10 or more pounds of water. That's the problem with the current all-the-rage, low carb diets—they are notorious glycogen depleters. And once you stop dieting, or go back to eating enough carbs, that water weight you lost so quickly will return just as fast.

A bane to beauty

Most people say they diet to look better. However, the "skin deep" aspect of beauty really takes a toll from dieting. Years of dieting causes the skin to lose its elasticity, which often results in stretch marks and premature wrinkles. And even your "crowning glory" may become less glorious. Remember—hair is protein, and many diets that fail to meet your protein needs can leave you with hair loss after just five to ten weeks. After years of dieting you can look forward to wrinkles and thinning hair, not to mention shrunken muscles, fatigue, and mood swings. Oh! And dieting diminishes beauty in another way: People who are constantly talking about or thinking about diets are just plain boring and depressing.

Bringing on bingeing

Ironically, diets set you up to do just the opposite: binge. The urge to binge is both psychological and physiological. The psychology is simple: we all crave what's

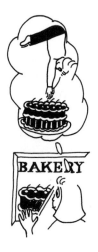

forbidden. No wonder, then, that after denying ourselves of certain foods or flavors long enough, we cave in and go for it with a vengeance!

But bingeing isn't brought on only by psychological cravings. Your hormones and brain are also likely to conspire against you if your calorie intake is so low that your body thinks it's starving. For instance, if your diet causes your blood sugar to drop too low, your brain may begin sending out signals (cravings) for foods high in sugar. You end up bingeing throughout the diet, which can be a source of great distress. Your self-esteem plummets and you compensate for the lapse by restricting your food intake even more.

Losing touch with your body's wisdom

In the best of all possible worlds, you could trust your body to tell you what you need, when you need it. But diets set up an artificial relationship between what your body needs and what your brain craves. Dieting messes up your hunger signals—after all, when you're dieting you're essentially eating less calories than you burn. So you're constantly feeling as if you haven't eaten enough, and forbidden (by your diet) to do anything about it.

Dieting can make real problems for you if you cook for other people as well as yourself. Since *they're* not on a diet, you end up facing temptation every time you cook a family meal. And sitting at the table with your cottage cheese on lettuce while they're enjoying big bowls of spaghetti can make you CRAZY!

In addition, the bingeing phenomenon described earlier contributes to confusing your body about what it needs. When you're feeling the psychological push of cravings for all the foods on the "forbidden" list, you're hardly likely to notice that what you *really* need are salads and cottage cheese!

Misplaced priorities

Let's face it: Dieting escalates the importance of food in your everyday life—you're always obsessing about the caloric value of the foods you've eaten and worrying about the number of calories in the food you are about to eat.

But for those of us who are raising kids, there's an even more insidious problem with the way that dieting can take over our lives. After all, we set an example for our children through our behavior. Nutritionists have long understood that the eating patterns of adults are actually formed in childhood. If we're obsessing about our food, therefore, we are also likely to pass our obsessions along to our children—especially our daughters.

Hurts the heart and other vital organs

Dieting can really put your heart and other vital organs under a lot of strain. If you're like many dieters, you probably diet for a couple of weeks, lose a few pounds, then go off the diet (and feel like you've failed). A few weeks later, you get right back on that diet rollercoaster and the cycle starts all over again. The on-again, off-again cycle ends up causing you to lose muscle—including heart muscle—and gain fat several times a year! That can cause real some real physical stress on your internal organs.

And if *that* isn't enough, some of the more extreme diets—not to mention eating disorders like anorexia—can cause even more stress! When your body weight gets too low, electrolytic imbalances can cause a dangerously low or irregular heartbeat! This is *not* something you want to fool around with!

Fertility problems

Body fat and femininity go hand in hand. Fat starts to accumulate in girls at puberty, coinciding with a genetically set clock. Estrogen is stored in fat and scientists now believe there is a minimum amount of fat necessary for the onset of menstruation.

In addition, females are genetically programmed to store more body fat than males—in order to sustain pregnancy and breast feeding. When you lose too much body fat through dieting, you can delay the onset of menstruation in adolescence, and diminish, or even *lose*, your ability to get pregnant later on.

Personality problems

If you've noticed a shorter concentration span while dieting, it's probably because your train of thought is interrupted by food fantasies, produced courtesy of the hypothalamus in the brain. But that's not all that dieting can do to affect your mood and personality. Dieting can cause you to tire more easily, it can cause insomnia, and it can even cause a loss of sex drive! This is because your brain's impulse is to conserve energy during what it perceives as periods of starvation. As a result, dieting makes you more susceptible to mental and physical depression.

Skews your "set point"

One of the main reasons diets don't work is because our bodies are genetically programmed to maintain a certain weight and a certain amount of body fat. This preprogrammed weight is called your set point. While scientists aren't yet sure *exactly* how set point is regulated, they do know that one of the control mechanisms is in the hypothalamus—a small structure deep within the brain that receives signals from your fat cells and works like a thermostat. When fat cells reach the genetically determined (set point) levels, the hypothalamus sends out fewer hunger signals. When fat cells are depleted, hunger signals are released.

Also part of the set-point regulating mechanism is your metabolic rate. When you diet, or when you don't get enough exercise, your metabolic rate—the rate at which you burn calories—is lowered. This has the effect of increasing your set point— which means you start getting hunger signals more often. Some studies indicate that yo-yo dieting also raises your set point, though the evidence isn't completely clear on this score. On the other hand, exercise raises your metabolism, which can push your set point down.

So if you begin to live a healthier lifestyle, your body will naturally adjust to its natural weight. If you have shot way past your set point, then a lifestyle without diets will enable you to lose some weight. If your body keeps coming back to a certain weight even though you are exercising, living a healthier lifestyle, and no longer starving and bingeing, this is where your set point is meant to be. It's a way your body tells you that this weight is healthy for you and genetically this is what is natural for you.

So Let's Do Away with Diets!

All these downsides to dieting should give you all the more reason to ditch the diets. And there *is* a better way to achieve a healthy weight. That "better way" is to get your body moving at a comfortable level and tune into your body for its own clues about hunger and fullness. The concepts in this book will show you how to be healthier and happier at *any* size. Either way, you come out winning and feeling better about yourself.

So what can you lose by trying this? Only your poor self-esteem, your attachment of your self-worth to the number on the bathroom scale. And think of all you have to gain! Confidence! Freedom! Think about it: No more starving yourself before facing weigh-in scales at the diet program. No more misery when the scales show you gained a measly 1/2 pound, or counterproductively "rewarding" yourself for a small weight loss by going to the doughnut shop. No more messing with cards or "contracts" or keeping score of your calorie count for every morsel you eat.

Top Ten Reasons to Give Up Dieting

Let's take a look—a la David Letterman—at the Council on Size and Weight Discrimination's (1996) top ten reasons to give up dieting:

- #10: Diets don't work.
- #9: Diets are expensive.
- #8: Diets are boring.
- #7: Diets don't necessarily improve your health.
- #6: Diets don't make you beautiful.
- #5: Diets are not sexy.
- #4: Diets can turn into eating disorders.
- #3: Diets can make you afraid of food.
- #2: Diets can rob you of energy.
- #1: Diets take a toll on your self-confidence.

Anyone who has joined a weight-loss group will find these Weigh-In Cheats familiar, I'm sure!

- You argue that the scale "just MUST be off by half a pound!"
- You eat no food at all until after weigh-in.
- You make up for the pre-weigh-in fasting by bingeing right after the meeting, or cheating for the next couple of days.
- You wear the lightest clothes you've got on weigh-in day—and strip off those clunky earrings, 'cause they might add an ounce or two to the scales!

And I'm not kidding about that Number One Reason! Learning to love and accept yourself just as you are will give you greater self-confidence, better health, and a sense of well-being that will last a lifetime.

HERSTORY

Freedom, *by Becky Chase*

I learned to throw up during my first year of college. It seemed like a good idea at the time. I could eat two brownies at dinner instead of one, and not have to worry about gaining weight. Those brownies were delicious! I even *lost* weight by the end of my freshman year—so much weight that my sisters told me I was too skinny. I loved that and believed they were just jealous.

The high of being skinny (and starved) was short lived, however. I went to work for a donut shop that summer—$1.25 an hour and all the donuts I could eat. I could eat a lot of donuts! My weight ballooned by 30 or 40 pounds that summer. That was the beginning of 18 long years of dieting and bingeing (although I gave up the vomiting after only a few years—it was too humiliating). Ironically, after graduating from college I ended up choosing a career in the field of nutrition!

After developing malnutrition from having lived, literally, on donuts that first summer, I eventually formed a real appreciation for the importance of healthy food, and entered a fanatical phase of eating only "natural" foods. But my "good food/bad food" way of thinking only deepened, and my self-esteem took a double beating whenever I slipped and pigged out on junk food: Not only was I eating "bad" food, I was now a "bad" dietitian, too.

My first real understanding that dieting does not fix compulsive overeating came from several years of running an obesity treatment program. This was one of the very-low-calorie, all-liquid diets that were so popular in the 1980s. Seeing the emotional swings my clients went through convinced me there was something wrong with—or at least missing from—the dieting picture. Their euphoria with being "thinner than ever before" quickly became despair when they almost inevitably gained the weight back during the refeeding and maintenance phases of the program, when they were allowed to go back to eating solid foods. We tried everything we could think of to help our clients understand the underlying emotional causes of their overeating, but their fantasies of fasting and losing gobs of weight made it cognitively and emotionally impossible for them to really address these issues. By the time they were back on real food, they were gaining weight and giving up.

I quit dieting, personally and professionally, after leaving that job. It was then that I was able to really face my own food and body issues and to truly know that dieting was not only a poor way to lose weight, it was also a negative process that was keeping my eating disorder alive. Dieting is something that I will never do again. The freedom I've attained from giving up dieting and recovering from compulsive overeating is too precious.

I would be lying if I didn't say it is sometimes tempting to once again focus on weight and dieting in my life—though my weight is stable and healthy, I am not thin by society's standards. But now I know that when I start feeling that way, I am really feeling something else—a sense of somehow just not being good enough, usually. Fantasies about dieting and being thin are now just signals that I am not feeling good about myself. I do not dwell there. Instead, I look inside and see what is out of place. Any pain I feel is correctly labeled and now I know where to look for help. *That* is freedom.

Making the Break

It comes to all of us, and often more than once: The "moment of truth," the facing up, the decision. People never forget the first time they decided to give up dieting. "I remember . . . " they will say, and then they'll go on to tell about how they started on a fresh path. Like them, you may find it necessary to repeat your commitment over and over to yourself before it becomes a reality. That's perfectly OK and normal. After all, by rejecting a ride on the diet rollercoaster, you've made one of those pivotal decisions in life—confronting and rejecting an old, destructive pattern.

But breaking a lifelong pattern is not easy. When you choose to alter a familiar lifestyle, be prepared: Interesting inner dialog will bubble up, sometimes helping you maintain your new choice, other times trying to sabotage it.

Keeping to your resolve to stay focused on this new, healthy journey may not always be easy, and you'll sometimes be tempted to slip back into your old ways. But there's something that can help strengthen your resolve. Take your initial decision and visualize it all shined up like a trophy. In your mind's eye, look at it when you need support to make the decisions that will come down the road. Mentally replay the events that led up to you taking action. If and when you fall back on old habits, don't give up on yourself. Instead, get up, dust off, remind yourself why you started and how you started—and get going again. Take note: this is not starting over, it's continuing from where you left off.

I hear stories all the time about the everyday courage and perseverance of former dieters who are embracing the diet-free, self-accepting decision for better health—

and you, too, will soon have your own personal and powerful story to draw on. To help you stay on track, here are a couple of key tips:

1. *Use Affirmations.* Affirmations are positive statements about yourself and your situation. They keep you motivated by affirming the progress you are making. For instance, you might say something like: "I like myself. I feel good about myself. I am going to have a great day." The more you say them, the more your affirmations will become true for you. They also help you to build up your self-esteem. Penny Muir, whose writings appear throughout this book, had this to say about affirmations: "As silly as I thought this was in the beginning it really was key to my success and it still helps me when I feel the chips are down."

I like myself!

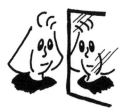

I am a worthwhile person!

2. *Use Confrontations.* When you feel yourself getting ready to slip back into an old, destructive pattern, build in a pause: Take time out to assess the situation and meet it head on—what we at HUGS call a "confrontation." Here's how confrontations work: Let's say that you catch yourself reaching for "comfort" food one evening because you're feeling bad about something that happened during the day. You're not really hungry, you just want to numb your feelings. With confrontation, you take a moment before rushing off to find something to eat. Instead, you let yourself sit with your feelings for as long as you can stand—whether that's a few minutes or even just a few seconds. Ask yourself: Why am I reaching for food? If, after you've taken this "time-out," you discover that you really *are* hungry, then fine—go for it. If you really *aren't* hungry, however, try thinking of alternatives to eating. Is there something else you can do instead?

I am going to have
a great day!

Perhaps talk to a friend? Take a quiet moment? Sip a cup of tea? These confrontations can be useful even if you're in the middle of a binge. It's *never* too late to take time out to stop, regain your control, and rethink your choices.

The Diet Free Option

If dieting is so destructive, what *can* you do to find, and achieve, a healthy weight? For one thing, you can start by listening to your body. It has a lot to tell you about how to find a healthy balance. Then you can switch your focus from dieting to nurturing yourself—and this includes healthier eating. Weight loss—if you need it—is sometimes a natural side effect of healthier eating.

Two thirds of all teenage girls in the United States have abnormal eating behavior, one half are severely undernourished, one third are smoking at least occasionally, one third are considering suicide, one fifth are overweight, and one tenth have potentially fatal eating disorders. (Source: *Afraid to Eat: Children and Teens in Weight Crisis*, Francie Berg, Healthy Weight Publishing Network, 2001, www.HealthyWeightNetwork. com).

Ten Steps Toward Losing the Diet Mentality

If you're just making the commitment to jump off the diet rollercoaster, you may need a little help in readjusting your attitudes toward food and eating.

Heather Wiebe Hildebrand, with whom I co-wrote a cookbook called *Tailoring Your Tastes* (1995), developed the following 10 tips to put you on a healthier path.

1. Eat when you are hungry and stop when you are full. This is all about throwing away your scales, diet sheets, and fat-gram counters and rediscovering your body's own message system. This is a skill that came naturally to you as a baby, and you can master it again. As a baby, when you were hungry, you ate, and when you were full, you stopped. As you grew up, however, you became more and more aware of the calories, food values, grams of fat, and all the other "shoulds" and "shouldn'ts" of eating. Eating became a very regimented task—you learned to eat foods because they were from the "right" food group or had the "right" number of calories. But if you're quitting the diet mentality, it's time to start listening to your body's signals for when to eat and when to stop.

2. Eat regularly—every 3–6 hours—when your body is physically hungry. Your body requires regular inputs of food for energy to

function optimally. Eating at irregular times or skipping meals can set you up for eating to excess when you finally do get around to having some food. A regular food intake actually increases your metabolic rate, which can have the added benefit of lowering your set point and thereby lowering the weight at which your body naturally tends to settle.

3. Start your day with breakfast. The old adage is true: "Breakfast is the most important meal of the day." But breakfast means more than a cup of coffee! In order to get both body and mind going in the morning, you need to feed them. A good breakfast will rev up your system up so that you're ready to function for the day, and it will get you through to your next meal.

4. Keep your carbs and proteins balanced. As a check for a healthy balance, learn to observe what's on your plate. Aim for two-thirds to three-fourths of the food on your plate to be carbohydrates, the rest protein. This balance will provide you with both the energy *and* the satiety you need to make it to the next meal or snack. The carbohydrates in foods such as bread, cereal, pasta, grains, fruit, starchy vegetables, and milk breaks down into sugar (glucose). When these foods are digested they produce the energy your body needs. Protein, on the other hand, is used in the body to build tissues. It also helps to slow down the digestion of the sugars from carbohydrates.

5. Throw away the concepts of "good" and "bad" food. As soon as you legalize *all* foods, you will be surprised how less often you crave the

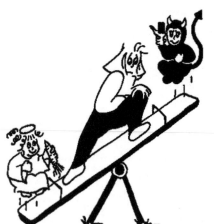

less nutritious ones. So taste, savor, and enjoy all foods to the fullest. When eating, pay attention to the experience—notice taste, texture, and aroma. The more attention you give your food, the more pleasure and satisfaction it will give you. You'll be surprised how often your body is satisfied with less when you give yourself the opportunity to enjoy the process, and the moment you legalized your favorite comfort foods, you regain power to choose to have them or not. And this approach works in reverse as well. The less attention and guilt you give to what you used to call a "bad" or "illegal" food, the less of it you need to be satisfied, and in some cases, the less comfort it provides—making it pointless to have anyway.

6. Be creative. Have fun with your new eating choices. By making changes and trying different foods and cooking techniques you can increase your enjoyment of eating and make mealtimes something to look forward to. For example, if you've always cooked your vegetables in water, try this for a change: Steam them to a crunchy tender stage with your favorite herb sprinkled on top. The new color, flavor, and texture will be a delight to your taste buds!

7. Find new ways to move your body. While you're learning to listen to your body's signals about hunger and fullness, start listening as well for what it's telling you about its need for activity or inactivity. You will be pleased to see how much better you feel both in body and soul when you start to move! But don't get me wrong—I'm not saying you have to spend hours at the gym or working out with fitness tapes. In fact, I say throw out the rules of fitness and simply start *moving*. Find activities that you love and do them, whether that activity is housework, gardening, yoga, or aerobics. Just moving your body for 20 minutes every day will have a *huge* impact on your health. As the popular slogan states: "Just do it!"

8. Take time out for yourself. In this busy world, many people—and especially women—end up spending all their time looking after other people. They look after their children, their significant others, their parents, their churches, their communities. Looking after *themselves* often becomes the last item on their "To Do" lists—and sometimes gets omitted entirely. But when you don't look after yourself, you become less effective, less efficient, and you have less fun. When you take time out for self-building, rest, and relaxation, on the other hand, you become rejuvenated. You need to look after yourself properly to be effective, happy, and healthy.

9. Take small steps when making changes. Ending a lifelong ride on the diet rollercoaster is a big change, and lasting change doesn't occur overnight. Instead, you're better off building up a series of smaller, more manageable changes. True, "take it slowly" seems like an alien concept in this "Instant Pudding" world where we seem to want everything to be done *yesterday*. But expecting instant change is

setting yourself up for failure. Your body likes what it "knows"—it will always want to go back to the familiar, especially when you are under stress. That's why, instead of trying to make big, overnight changes in your lifestyle, you're better off taking small, gradual steps.

10. Enjoy the process! Making a change in your lifestyle can be overwhelming, and if you move too quickly or if you don't give your body a chance to adapt and incorporate the changes you may find that you don't enjoy the process. And if you don't enjoy the process, you won't keep doing it. So whenever you find yourself feeling overwhelmed with the process of change, take a step back. Listen to your body. It has a lot to tell you about finding a healthy balance.

The Label Trap, *by Christie Keating*

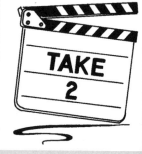

"I can't do this. It's too hard. I'm not cut out for this. The stress is too much. I quit."

These thoughts pass through my mind often, and not only when I'm deep in thought . . . they creep in on me all day. In other words, I'm an all-or-nothing thinker. But I've come to understand how debilitating this kind of thinking can be. How it closes off my options, thought patterns, and growth. It saps me of energy, leaves my head space cloudy and unsure, tugs at my confidence and self-esteem, and creates frustration and anxiety.

I seem to be able to only think in black and white with no shades of gray. The diet mentality is very much all or nothing. Having accepted the HUGS philosophy into my life, I've been able to see lots of "gray" around issues of food and physical activity. How come this freedom of thought hasn't wandered into the rest of my life?

Last week I was ready to throw in the towel. Single parenting, starting a business, and a looming court battle over child support had left me feeling pretty low. How can I be a successful entrepreneur if I have to be a full-time parent? How can I be a full-time parent and a successful entrepreneur if my financial base gets shattered? How can I be all of this? Do all of this?

Part of me wanted to close the door of my business. After all, it costs money and time to start up, so if I quit, then money and time stays with me. I even thought that maybe now would be a good time for the children to stay with their father. That would settle the parenting and monetary anxiety. Thinking this way dragged me even farther down. I was not allowing myself to think of options, to look at the long term. I was reaching out for the "quick fix."

I know in my heart that I want to live with my kids and that I love my work. If I loosen up my way of thinking, I will be able to see what options are out there that will let me keep what I love. But phrases like "have to" and "should" limit me right away. The small, gradual changes that I made about food and physical activity have become part of me, so maybe now it's time to look at other areas of my life and apply the same principals: reflection, knowledge, and small, gradual changes.

Because I've labeled myself as an "all or nothing" thinker, however, I've reinforced that message over and over again. So now it's time to find another label. One that is more "gray" and forgiving. How about just "Christie"?

An International Perspective

Before we move on, let me share with you these observations from a long-time proponent of the diet-free lifestyle—Wendyl Nissen. She's the former editor of *New Zealand Woman's Weekly*, the largest-circulation magazine in New Zealand. Her comments, appearing here with the kind permission of the magazine, first appeared in the May 5, 1997 issues. What she has to say is very much on target, and shows that the movement away from dieting has taken on a truly international scope!

> I was alarmed to read the other morning that women's magazines are being blamed for the unhealthy state of New Zealanders because we print "fad junk diets." "Well!" I exclaimed over my cup of tea. My pile of clippings on the bed had a swift addition and I was off to the office to do battle with the National Heart Foundation's Dr. Boyd Swinburn—the perpetrator of these comments. If there's one thing I'm strict on as an editor it's not running diets. . . .

> The reason I don't like diets is because of a deep-seated resentment for having spent my adolescence in the seventies—the diet decade. From my earliest memory, my mother was on a diet, and at high school all my friends were on diets. All around me people were turning orange from eating too many carrots! Yet somehow it became acceptable as part of our culture. Don't like yourself? Then diet.

I was unusually skinny as a teen but, amazingly, still felt the peer pressure to go on diets. Out went my naturally healthy eating habits and in came cravings that had never bothered me before. In those days we were all fuelled by the diets in magazines. It will take years for women to get over diets because health is still not a top priority—while body shape is. I'm still constantly astounded to find myself standing next to slim professional women who make a huge fuss about not eating or drinking because they are "trying to lose some weight." These women are tiny and I wonder what kind of message they give the women who work for them.

The real message we could be giving each other is high self-esteem. We could be learning to live with our bodies and enjoying them. Imagine if we all woke up one morning and looked in the mirror and liked what we saw. As women, we could probably spend more time encouraging each other to get some exercise than we spend urging each other to go on a diet. We could also tell each other how beautiful we look—we don't do enough of that. Next time someone near you looks fabulous, tell them, it really doesn't hurt.

Taking It Deeper

- **On: The Ugly Side of Dieting**

  1. Discuss the points brought out in this article on why not to diet. Do you agree with them?

- **On: Top Ten Reasons to Give up Dieting**

  1. Discuss the "Top Ten" reasons for giving up dieting as given in this chapter. Do you have reasons to add to this list?

- **On: Freedom**

  1. Becky Chase writes "Fantasies about dieting and being thin are now just signals that I am not feeling good about myself. I do not dwell there. Instead, I look inside and see what is out of place." Do you have "size" fantasies as well? Examine them and discuss what they may really be saying to you.

  2. Using your examination of "size" fantasies from the question above, discuss how you can constructively work through them, as Becky has done.

- **On: Making the Break**

  1. Describe the process that you went through to give up dieting. Include a discussion of any relapses, why they may have occurred, and how you have overcome them.

  2. Come up with a few positive statements—affirmations—that will reflect your situation to keep your life in balance and in perspective.

  3. In the HUGS philosophy, confrontation means meeting a situation head on and dealing with the causes of your feelings. Discuss ways in which you can use the confrontation technique to overcome the urge to use food inappropriately—as a comforter, for example.

- **On: Ten Steps Towards Losing the Diet Mentality**

  1. Over the next several days, try to incorporate at least one of these steps into your daily life. As you begin to feel comfortable with one, add another—and reward your progress by checking off the steps as you feel you have mastered them.

  2. If you discover that one or more of the steps is really hard for you to master, try to apply the "confrontation" technique to examine what the difficulty might be. Discuss ways in which the step can be broken down into smaller, easier stages.

- **On: The Label Trap**

  1. How would you label yourself? Are you an all-or-nothing thinker, one that sees things as black and white? Or are you able to put some shades of gray into the way you view food, activity, and life situations? Discuss the steps you might take to make the transition out of the label trap.

  2. Pick a situation from your own life and contrast the two ways of looking at them—first, through the all-or-nothing approach, and second, through the approach that acknowledges "shades of gray." How do the two ways of looking at the situation compare? Which provides the most constructive, positive experience?

3. When people experience a momentary lapse or setback, many
    people are tempted to give up altogether. Discuss the reasons that
    this might happen, and how you might overcome such a temptation.
    Does Christie's experience with breaking out of all-or-nothing
    thinking provide insights that might be helpful in your own life?

- **On: An International Perspective**

    1. Discuss the impact that women's magazines, the fashion industry,
        insurance companies, the medical community, and others have had
        on shaping the diet mentality that permeates society's definition of
        "healthy." How can these influences be challenged?

    2. When was the last time you were given a compliment? How well did
        you accept it? How did it make you feel?

    3. When was the last time you told someone else she or he looked
        fabulous? How was the compliment received? How did it seem to
        make the recipient feel?

Ditching the Diet Dialogue 3

Breaking Loose
Change Your Brain
Buddy Up!
  Untangle yourself from the diet web
  Passion ignited
This Really Works: A Before and After
  Diet mentality quizzes, compared
  Making it meaningful
Taking It Deeper

L et's say you've accepted that diets don't work; that you've come to realize that *you* haven't failed at dieting—the diets failed you. So how come, even though you've made a commitment to living without diets, you still have diet talk rattling around in your brain?

The answer is simple: Because diet talk—and the diet mentality—is inescapable in this society. It surrounds us. It comes from parents, friends, relatives, and strangers. We're all guilty of thinking of food in destructive ways: food is either a "bad guy" or a comforter and friend. It's never simply a healthy source of nourishment.

Once you've clued into this invasion of your thought processes and decisions, you'll be amazed to discover how it's always cropping up to rob you of many of life's potential pleasures. For many, dieting is a system of control that can rob us of the ability to enjoy even the simplest of activities. Even *talking* about diets reflects that element of control—so much "diet talk" includes phrases like: "I didn't exercise, so I can't have that donut," "I have to eliminate sweets, or I can't wear that swimsuit," and so on. Diets, in other words, are all about punishments, with only the occasional reward thrown in to keep you going.

A lifestyle without diets, on the other hand, offers freedom. It offers you the opportunity to enjoy the present moment. It encourages you to adopt an attitude of experimentation and discovery about the food you eat and the activities you enjoy. It teaches you to rediscover your body's wisdom about how much and what types of food you need for your natural level of activity.

Breaking Loose

So you've decided that you want the advantages of a diet-free lifestyle—but how do you go against this ever-present, pro-dieting tide? My answer comes in three parts:

- Develop a sense of humor about society's dieting mentality.
- Rekindle your awareness of your body's own wisdom of its needs.
- Develop a strong support system that reinforces your diet-free lifestyle.

Your first step toward a lifestyle without diets is to be a diet-mentality detective! The world's on a diet, and it shows up everywhere: in commercials and advertisements, posters, magazine headlines. Take a good look around you and *laugh* at the silliness you see. After all, the alternative is to let that mentality creep into your *own* perceptions. So that's your next step—to become aware of just how much your eating behaviors have been colored by the images you're bombarded with every day. One way to increase your awareness is through keeping up a conscious running dialogue in your head, chronicling your reactions to food and food cues. At HUGS I encountered one participant who did just that—she shared with us the running dialogue she had been keeping up for a single week. I bet many of her thoughts sound familiar:

- I think I let myself get too hungry.
- I tend to overeat when the family's all here. I guess I'm celebrating.
- I just ate that treat because the others were eating. Didn't even taste it. Excitement usually takes my appetite for a while but I usually make up for it later.
- Why do I always want to eat more than I should?
- I'm surprised I wasn't all that hungry and didn't eat all that much, just the wrong things.
- Why couldn't I just wait till supper?
- That ham tasted good, although I felt guilty about too much fat on it.
- Craving sweets but there's nothing in the house.
- I'm afraid I've eaten too much—but it tasted so good I couldn't resist.
- I feel guilty for eating so much pasta.
- The comfort foods appealed to me today. I told myself I was buying them for the children, but I really wanted them for myself.
- I had two and a half donuts with my lunch and feel out of touch and into denial.
- I bought an ice cream bar and strawberry drink; it was good and I'm not even feeling guilty.
- Stuffed myself at supper—didn't manage to stop myself in time. Whenever this happens I feel ashamed of myself.
- I'm feeling frustrated by the pain of a friend's divorce—I tend to absorb other people's pain. That's probably why I ate half of that small package of candies.
- Preparing food for company, I find myself resenting having to rush, and wondering how I'll get everything done in time.
- I understand all the ins and outs of a healthy diet but I'm a bit of a rebel. My problem goes deeper than what I eat.

As my friend's experience shows, you'll be amazed at the kind of things you'll find yourself thinking when you start becoming aware of your thoughts about food!

Change Your Brain

Whew, huh? If that list was like the sound track in *your* brain, it's time to change the tape! One good way to do this is to look carefully at the words associated with dieting: You'll discover that they're all *negative*:

Diet Talk

should/should not   adhere

comply

only   need

prescribe   deprived

illegal   know

hate   tell

allow   control

must/must not

forbidden   have to

Notice how all those words are restrictive? They all set limits on your choices in life. But how about replacing them with freedom words from this next list?

Freedom Words

could   enable   examine

feel

in tune   encourage

study   reflect

experience   discover   identify

might

explore   empower

enjoy

love   reflect

Once you've familiarized yourself with the
restrictive words from diet talk, start
observing how often they crop up in the
conversations around you—and even in
your *own* language. Diet dialogue sets an
agenda you don't want to buy into any
longer. Fight back with freedom words.
When you find yourself saying "I should,"
replace it with "I prefer to" or "I could."
Instead of saying "I must," try "I'll explore
it." The change in words will help you
build a change in your whole attitude!

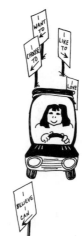

Still, the diet mentality will creep back
into your thought patterns every once in
awhile—you've been living with it all your life, after all. The secret is to be able to
identify it when it happens. Then you can fight back.

Buddy Up!

Making changes in your lifestyle can be difficult if you try to go it alone. The
solution: Seek out help for the journey. When you are with a supportive group or
buddy, you can tap into a powerful process. With a friend, it's easier to laugh at the
silliness of "It tasted good although I felt guilty about too much fat on it." Alone,
you might fall back into the misery of "I'm ashamed of myself."

Change is difficult, especially if you've spent years on the diet rollercoaster.
Laughter, shared with supportive friends, lightens the load. Harness the energy of
others, and be there for *them* when they need *your* support. The strength you receive
from this shared experience will make your own quest for change easier.

A HUGS support group in Winnipeg, Canada really understands the destructive
effect of the diet mentality. They place a strong emphasis on digging out diet
thinking and replacing those negative comments with some meaningful group
guidance. Whenever individual group members expose "diet mentality" in their
comments, group members are always willing to provide guidance on switching
over to "freedom thinking." Here are some actual comments and group
responses—along with a few of my own thoughts and background to help round out
the point.

Untangle Yourself from the Diet Web		
Diet Mentality Comments	*Responses from Support Group*	*My Guidance*
I ignore my "cravings" and instead I usually eat "good" food but I really don't enjoy it.	Appreciate and enjoy your cravings. By ignoring your cravings, you'll end up eating more of other foods.	Ask yourself why do you have the cravings to begin with? Did you skip a meal? Are you under-eating? Is it hormonal? Address these issues and if your craving is there because of hunger, then eating a substantial snack or meal will make it go away. If it doesn't go away, then try eating what you crave, but savor every mouthful; otherwise the craving will just build and all of a sudden the entire cookie jar is empty. Paying attention and tasting and enjoying your food without feeling guilty allows you to be satisfied with less.
I'm not a breakfast eater. I'm usually starving by noon.	Breakfast kick-starts your day. It provides energy and keeps you alert. Then the chance of overeating later is reduced.	Years of skipping breakfast have taught your body to not expect it. You can retrain your body to want breakfast in just a few days. Note that it's quite normal to be hungry at lunch time whether or not you have had breakfast, but by having breakfast you'll experience normal hunger at lunch and dinner rather than being ravenous.

Untangle Yourself, cont'd . . .		
I'm going out for a big dinner. I won't eat all day so I can really pig out.	Try to have a snack or something before you head out. You can still enjoy the meal without going over the point of feeling comfortably full.	You want to come to the meal comfortably hungry so that you can enjoy your food, eat it slowly, and take in the entire experience: atmosphere, companions, and so on. If you don't eat all day you'll end up being so hungry that you don't actually taste your food: You'll be gobbling it down to satisfy your voracious appetite.
I'll accept myself when I lose 20 pounds first.	You have to accept yourself as you are *today*.	For many, finding self-acceptance is a long process that takes time. To help it along, practice turning your negative thinking around by using positive affirmations. With self-acceptance will come a greater ability to make small changes in your lifestyle to become healthier no matter *what* your size. No more feeling bad about yourself! Freedom!!
I'll have more self-esteem, confidence, and self-worth with weight loss.	You can have all those wonderful qualities without weight loss.	If your self-esteem, confidence, and self-worth are only based on weight loss, it is short lived and will yo-yo along with your weight. Isn't it time to detach your self-worth from your weight and find other areas to bring out these qualities? When you stop putting so much

Untangle Yourself, cont'd . . .

		energy into weight loss, you will be able to channel your newfound energies into more productive areas that will truly increase your confidence, self-worth, and self-esteem. Go with it!
I weigh myself daily to see how I'm progressing.	You don't need to check the scales to see how you're progressing.	Ask yourself what happens when you use the scale to measure progress. Does checking the scales make you feel better about yourself when you lost weight? Maybe, but how about when the weight comes back? You don't feel so good about yourself, right? You might even feel like a failure. Free yourself from such negatives and learn to key into new ways of measuring success through changes in your attitude and behavior.
I bought some clothes a size smaller than I wear, to be an incentive to lose weight.	You just spent money that will not benefit you. Buy clothes that fit you as you are today.	If you buy clothes that are too small, you feel bad that you can't get into them. Feeling bad about yourself can lead to over-eating, defeating the entire purpose. Buy something that looks good on you *now*, and see how it affects your behavior and attitude in a positive way.

Untangle Yourself, cont'd . . .		
I have to eat low-fat foods to be healthier. But I don't enjoy eating them and usually "pig out" later on.	Enjoy the foods you love. Going low-fat suddenly will be a shock to your system. Try adding low-fat foods slowly.	The nondiet process gives your taste buds a chance to adjust. In time, you'll actually find yourself choosing to eat foods that are healthier for you because you prefer them.
I'm not dieting any more. Instead, I'm on a "lifestyle eating program" and it tells me what I should be eating and what I should stay away from.	It's a diet in disguise. People hate the term "diet," so diet companies are coming up with new buzz words so they won't turn people away.	Diet companies are very cleverly repackaging their message when they tell people they can eat whatever they want. But they still make you count fat grams, fiber grams, and so forth. The latest wrinkle is the new "point system." But this approach tunes out any consideration of your body's actual needs.
I'm very obese and haven't been able to go to a restaurant because the chairs have arms and I can't fit in them. I have to lose weight to be able to enjoy life.	Before you dine out simply ask the restaurant for a sturdy chair without arms. They will be glad to accommodate you. If they can't provide a chair, go to a restaurant that *will* provide one.	Stop putting your life on hold just because of your size. Choose places that work for you—where you feel comfortable. The diet-free lifestyle teaches you how to be more assertive so that you *do* feel comfortable, no matter what your current size.
I've been trying this approach, but I feel discouraged and don't see any weight loss.	It takes time, so have patience with yourself. After years of being on diets, old habits die hard. Talk about your frustrations. And remember, your body may be at its set point.	Remember that while dieting sometimes results in quick weight loss, in most cases there's quick weight gain as well, later on. Dieting is artificial because it does not allow you to listen to your body, which is why the yo-yo

Untangle Yourself, cont'd . . .

		syndrome occurs. With a diet-free approach, on the other hand, you are listening to your body, nourishing it, and enjoying the way your body moves —and your body adjusts to where it is naturally meant to be. For some that may mean weight loss, for others it may mean weight stabilization or even some weight gain, as your body finds its proper weight.
My fiance said I'll have to lose weight before he marries me.	If he can't accept and love you as you are, then it's a sign for you to move on. Life will be miserable with this person.	Ask yourself why you are staying with someone who makes you feel bad about yourself. There may be underlying reasons of sabotage here and you may need some professional counseling to help you move on. How can you love someone who only loves you conditionally and not for who you really are?
I'll be happier, more healthier, slimmer.	You can be happy and healthier at any size.	Nondiet thinking may be a big leap for some. To help you actually accept yourself, reflect back as to whether being slimmer actually did make you healthier. Ask yourself, were you preoccupied with food and weight all the time? Were you undereating to maintain this lower weight? As a result, did you binge

Untangle Yourself, cont'd . . .		
		more often? Were you actually happier when you were slimmer? Did all of your problems just vanish because of your slimmer size? Did other problems surface? Do these questions indicate improved health? Don't think so.

It's clear that breaking free of the diet mentality is an important step toward jumping off the diet rollercoaster. If you're finding it hard to break free, however, take heart. We all have to struggle with the old patterns of thinking that we grew up with, but lots of us have ultimately succeeded. You can too.

HERSTORY

Passion Ignited, *by Shelley McDonald*

In the foreword to the book *You Count, Calories Don't*, Rena A. Mendelson says: "The pages of this book should be read over and over again until the principles have been gradually integrated into a lifestyle change." That is what I have done over the last two years and very gradually, but steadily, I have changed many poor habits and negative mindsets, and though the process continues, I feel that I have been liberated from the obsessiveness of the diet mentality. I wake up in the mornings looking forward to living the day, no longer concerned with thoughts of what I can eat and what I can't, and what jeans I can squish into. I eat when I'm hungry, eat what I want, and stop when I'm full, monitoring myself only by how I feel. And I feel good!

It's so simple really, and yet society has so complicated it. And we are all susceptible. Even after becoming vocally anti-diet, over Christmas holidays I found myself eating continually. Aware that it wasn't hunger, I finally realized it was the diet mentality, insidious as it is. For all dieters know that you binge on all the goodies in December and in January, you diet! It was a good reminder for me. I forgot that too much crappy food makes you feel crappy and that overeating Christmas dinner leaves you feeling lethargic and lousy. Instead of going to play games with your friends or going for a walk with your family, you can't get off the couch. And I had forgotten how awful it is to feel out of control around food. We are talking quality of life here.

I just want to encourage all of you to continue with the process, put food back in its proper perspective. Listen to your body and respond to it. Remember that good health is your right and privilege.

This Really Works: A Before and After

Here's how one woman is faring in her liberation from the diet mentality. Like you are doing in this book, she measures her progress with the Diet Mentality Quiz that you took in Chapter One.

Sandra Olafson went through the HUGS at Home program and now says that living without diets has been a life-changing experience. "For the first time in my life, I haven't been preoccupied with the scale or comparing myself with other women my age or younger. I'm not depressed by thoughts like 'It's almost summer and I've got to get thin in the next three months.' I have replaced the idea of getting thin with a focus on health. Being thin is not important anymore."

After six months of working the program, Sandra wanted to see how far she had progressed in that time, so she went back and retook the Diet Mentality Quiz. Sandra's changing perceptions show up in a before-and-after comparison of her quiz scores—looking at how her current answers differed from the ones she gave at the start of the program. Just look at how her diet mentality has changed!

Diet Mentality Quizzes, Compared			
Score: 1 = Always; 2 = Very Often; 3 = Often; 4 = Sometimes; 5 = Rarely; 6 = Never			
Question Number	Before	After	
1.	3	5	I am unhappy with myself the way I am.
2.	2	4	I am preoccupied with a desire to be thinner.
3.	4	6	I weigh myself several times a week.

Question Number	Before	After	
4.	4	6	I am more concerned with the number on the scale than my overall sense of well-being.
5.	3	5	I think about burning up calories when I exercise.
6.	4	4	I am out of tune with my body for natural signals of hunger and fullness.
7.	3	4	I eat for other reasons than physical hunger.
8.	2	4	I eat too quickly, not taking time to focus on my meal and taste, savor and enjoy my food.
9.	3	4	I fail to take time for activities for myself.
10.	3	4	I fluctuate between periods of sensible, nutritious eating and out-of-control eating.
11.	3	5	I give too much time and thought to food.
12.	6	6	I tend to skip meals, especially early in the day, so I can "save up" my food for one big feast.
13.	3	6	I engage in all-or-nothing thinking.
14.	2	3	I try to be all things to all people.
15.	3	4	I strive for perfection in my life.
16.	3	4	I criticize myself for not achieving my goals.

"Before" Total: 51 + 4 = 55
"After" Total: 74 + 4 = 78

Making it meaningful

It's clear from Sandra's before-and-after scores that she's come a long way from her old diet mentality. And she's gone *way* up in her self-esteem. Just look at the change in her responses to questions 1, 4, 9, and 16! In all four of these areas, which are directly related to how good she feels about herself and how well she treats herself, she's gained at least one point—in a couple of cases she's actually gone up *two* whole points! Clearly she's making great progress in developing a positive self-image.

And when it comes to the questions that directly relate to her attitudes and behaviors toward food, she shows an equally impressive progress. She has obviously learned to reduce her tendency to eat too much or for the wrong reasons, and she is more consistent in eating sensibly and nutritiously. Thoughts of food no longer obsess her.

In addition, she has made real progress in overcoming the self-defeating attitudes that come with the diet mentality. She is definitely learning not to judge her personal growth by such artificial measures as the bathroom scale, and she has markedly reduced her focus on thinness as a goal. She has also learned to be more understanding of herself and her limits—she is clearly learning to cut back on the perfectionist, all-or-nothing attitude that so easily leads to feelings of failure, and she is learning not to be so self-critical.

Sandra is truly an on-going success story. You can be too.

Taking It Deeper

- **On: Change Your Brain**

    1. Pay attention to your own vocabulary. When you catch yourself using phrases that employ restrictive, diet-mentality words, practice substituting the freedom phrases of the diet-free lifestyle.

    2. Diet talk is very deeply ingrained in our society. Tune into the diet talk around you and in your head, then turn it around. As you become more confident, you may decide to speak up and make a difference in turning around society's diet thinking and diet talk.

- **On: Untangle Yourself From the Diet Web**

    1. Learning to counter diet talk and thoughts with nondiet responses is the key to living a diet-free lifestyle. Work through the diet mentality comments and support-group responses in this chapter's chart. Try to come up with an explanation for why the nondiet response works. See if you can come up with your own suggestions

for nondiet responses and come up with a few situations where you can use them.

2. One example in the chart mentions "diets in disguise." Give examples of some of the diets in disguise that you've noticed lately. Explain why they appear to be nondiet and yet they are truly just repackaging the same diet message of shoulds and shouldn'ts of eating. Give examples how, like traditional diets, these new programs set a person up for failure.

3. From the responses (both the HUGS group and my own) look for examples of how taking action can help a person get on with his or her life. How can taking action make you feel good?

4. Why is the sentence "You haven't failed . . . diets failed you" so powerful in helping you to let go of the false premise that diets work?

5. Identify personal situations that encourage your unhealthy relationship with food (over- *and* under-eating), as well as situations that send you running for the comfort of food rather than friend, or swearing off "bad" food. Make a list of the situations you have identified.

6. Make a list of non-food ways of dealing with crises that work for you. Examples might include taking a bubble bath, reading, walking, telephoning a friend, or immersing yourself in a hobby.

- **On: Passion Ignited**

1. Consider Shelley's journey and her recommendations for handling holiday time. Do you recognize any suggestions and attitude changes that are appropriate for your own situation?

- **On: This Really Works: A Before and After**

1. Compare Sandra's "before" and "after" scores. Take a moment now to retake your own Diet Mentality quiz and compare it to your original scores to see how you, too, have begun to move forward. While you're back in Chapter One to take the quiz, review the chart called "Your State of Change." Have you made progress in improving your own readiness for change?

Lose Weight and Call Me In the Morning

4

What's Up, Doc?
Converting My Doctor
Me and My Non-Number
Standing Up For Your Rights
So *That's* Why He Wants Me To Lose Weight

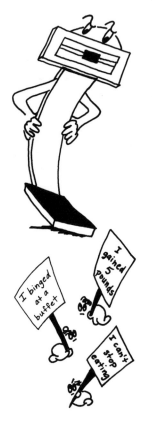

J ust hop on the scales.

For many of us, those are the five most dreaded words to be heard at the doctor's office, closely followed by, "You really need to go on a diet and lose weight."

If you hear these words routinely when you go in for a check-up, it's time for a little doctor re-education (or dietitian, or nurse practitioner, or any other health-care professional). As many of you already know, the nondiet message still hasn't reached many of the people working in the field of healthcare. So what do you say to your doctor about your newfound, diet-free attitude toward weight? Read on—this chapter will give you the ammunition you need, so that by your next doctor's visit you'll know what to say.

The more you know about the diet-free lifestyle, the better chance you have of successfully educating the health professionals who provide you with your care. The more confident you are in your new lifestyle, shifts in attitude, and changed behavior, the easier it is to convince your doctor that these changes, and not the numbers on the scale, are the true signs of success. And that's the message you want to convey: When weight loss is the barometer of health, and diets are the only way to get there, you're likely to end up even heavier down the road—*not* a good place to be.

But don't expect it to be easy to convince a traditional, diet-minded doctor to change her approach overnight. Doctors can become set in their ways. They can also be very persuasive in trying to bring you back to *their* way of thinking. You'll have to stay strong and refuse to buy into the suggestion that one more diet is what you need. Instead, let your health-care professional know that you're committed to a gradual lifestyle change. Explain how fine-tuning your eating and activity habits frees you from being preoccupied with food and weight.

What's Up, Doc?

Whenever health professionals prescribe a weight loss diet for you, first find out *why* they want you to lose weight. Some—thank goodness a minority—will actually suggest weight loss purely for the sake of vanity. That sort of suggestion can simply be ignored. On the other hand, if weight loss is prescribed in order to improve your health, you can use this as an opportunity to educate your health-care professional. The stage is set for you to re-educate your caregivers. Here's how to do it:

- Talk about how you have learned from personal experience that diets not only aren't a permanent solution to weight loss, but often end up making you heavier.

- Explain that health has come to mean something more to you than simply becoming slimmer.

- Explain the changes you are making in your life in order to improve your health.

- Be assertive with your observations about your own progress, and explain why it is no longer based on the numbers on the scale. Many doctors and other health professionals are still under the assumption that if you make healthy changes in your lifestyle, you must surely lose weight. If they see no weight loss, they assume that you are probably *not* making the changes you claim. Explain how, sometimes, weight loss takes time, and sometimes it doesn't happen at all—improvements in health, like lower cholesterol and improved blood pressure and blood sugar levels, aren't necessarily accompanied by loss of weight!

- Remind your health professional that, sometimes, improvements in diet and exercise can result in weight *gain*, as you are increasing muscle while you are losing fat.

- Talk about how you are increasing your activity levels and how activity has become a fun part of life.

- Tell about how you are retraining your taste buds so that you now enjoy foods that contain less fat and sugar.

- Emphasize that you are making these changes gradually, altering your taste preferences so that you don't develop cravings for "forbidden" foods and later binge on them. Explain how this helps you avoid the yo-yo cycle that dieting has set you off on in the past.

- Explain how the yo-yo trend actually increased your risk of heart disease and diabetes (two main reasons why physicians encourage weight loss).

- Talk about how you are learning to balance your food choices, encouraging your metabolism to rev up so that you stay full longer.
- Tell your health professional how good you feel, both mentally and physically, since you've stopped dieting and started focusing on being healthier.
- Finish by explaining that you have made a conscious choice to strive for gradual changes, because you know that they will last.

After hearing you work through these points, any responsible health-care professional will recognize that you are indeed striving for improved health, that you are making your own decisions, and that these decisions are based on a sound, health-conscious program. But some doctors are set in their ways. If your doctor does not accept your decisions, maybe it's time to change doctors. It's your choice—you can stay with a non-supportive doctor, or you can seek out one who understands your decision to work with your body and to ignore society's image of "normal" at the expense of your health.

And health professionals often *do* come around to accepting a nondiet way of life. For instance, here's what a dietitian wrote to me:

> I realized that an alternative [to dieting] was needed when a client came to see me about two years ago. I proceeded to start with the traditional diet, and she immediately said, "Look, I'll be honest. I've been on every diet in the book and I weigh more than ever." The more I got to know this client and work with her, the more my own mindset has changed. Instead of working on weight loss as a goal, we worked on improving health and being more healthy, physically and emotionally.

> This client has been so successful it is astounding. What amazes me is that her doctor did not see her success since there was very little weight loss involved. She has since changed doctors and has found a more understanding, accepting, and enlightened doctor.

So, remember the facts:

- Diets don't work.
- Pounds may be lost but they always come back.

The failure rate of dieting is between 96 and 98 percent, according to Dr A. Feinstein of the American College of Physicians and many other leading health professionals.

No wonder more and more of us are beginning to insist "You haven't failed at the diet—the diet has failed *you!*"

You *can* enlist your health-care professional's attitude toward dieting. Ask Heather —she knows.

Converting My Doctor, *by Heather Wiebe Hildebrand*

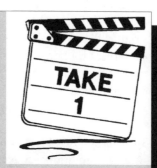

The term "health" confuses me.

What does healthy mean? Who decides if I am healthy? Do I? Does my doctor? Does society? Is health something that just happens because of fate or is it something that you work hard at achieving?

Some of the most confusing messages about health that I have received over the years have come from the medical profession. As a child and young adult I was taught to implicitly trust in the health profession. They allegedly knew what was best for me and would guide me to become as healthy as I possibly could be. Today we are told "buyer beware" in all services, even in the health profession.

In the past, physicians told me to lose weight at almost any cost. I was put on very low calorie diets and on intense exercise regimens. I was to become healthier by being thinner. I always got thinner, but I always gained the weight back after completing the process. Was my doctor actually helping me to become a healthier person or was it "weight loss at all costs" thinking?

My greatest fear after I started participating in the HUGS program was going to see my physician. My doctor seemed to see thinness as the only route to health, but I no longer agreed. Instead, I hoped to change my lifestyle habits and stop focusing on weight loss. The gradual life changes I was implementing didn't result in instant weight loss. Research has shown that my feast-or-famine patterns of eating had probably increased my health risks due to constant weight fluctuations. I thought for a long time about what health and healthiness meant to me, and I was learning to live a healthier lifestyle gradually. The key was the gradual nature of the process. I wanted to get off of the diet rollercoaster forever. I wanted the change to last a lifetime.

The day came when I needed to go and see my physician. How would my doctor and I resolve our differences? Our goal was similar—we both wanted me to become a healthier person—but the routes we followed were different. With a quaking heart I entered the office.

Regardless of my ailment or complaint, my doctor would always weigh me and suggest weight loss. This visit was no different. My doctor suggested I should lose weight by cutting out all fat and exercising religiously every day. Tremulously I explained that my lifestyle had areas that needed improvement. I told of how I was gradually making changes. I was changing my eating, activity, and attitude patterns. I told the doctor about the HUGS plan for better health and how this approach was helping me make lasting changes. I talked about my past history of weight fluctuations on various eating and exercise regimens and suggested that this actually increased my health risks more than stabilizing at a higher weight would.

Concluding that I felt I was making positive changes towards a healthier lifestyle, I asked for additional suggestions on achieving my goal. The physician's response was supportive and encouraging. I am not sure that my physician is totally sold on the process, because he still identifies weight loss as the most important goal. However, he now recognizes that the process I have chosen is sensible, feasible, and healthy. My doctor now realizes that diets haven't helped me achieve this goal in the past, and that even though diets have helped me to lose some weight, the weight has always returned. It was time to change the approach. I want the changes in my life to be permanent, not just another diet that I will get tired of and discard.

You'll notice that Heather didn't just march into her doctor's office and refuse his advice. She took the time to explain her position, in detail. That's key. And it's key for another reason—it helps you to strengthen your *own* commitment to the diet-free lifestyle. Just hearing yourself telling someone else about how this new way of living works can be immensely empowering.

Me And My Non-Number, *by Christie Keating*

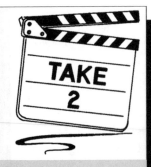

My friend Mary was a regular visitor to her bathroom scale. Her outlook for the day was formed by the number on the scale. By participating in HUGS, she was able to shed this attachment, however, and she moved her scale from its prominent position in the kitchen to a box in the storage unit of her apartment. There it stayed until International No-Diet Day, when it was recycled.

This was very liberating for Mary, but alas, she was soon tested. Mary was due for her annual physical, and we all know what *that* means: "step on the scale, please." Well, she called to tell me of her experience—and how *positive* it was!

When the nurse asked her to get on the scale she replied "I do not weigh myself anymore," and proceeded to explain the HUGS philosophy and how freeing it was to not be fixated on her weight. The nurse explained that she needed this number for her file, so Mary obliged her, and honored herself, by backing onto the scale and asking the nurse not to tell her the number—that it had no meaning for her! Her voice, as she told me this, reflected her immense pleasure at having asserted herself, and we both had quite a laugh at her "rear view" approach to the scale.

Coincidentally, my own physical was two days later. I was fairly certain, given the fact that this was my first visit with this doctor, that I would be asked my weight as well. It had been so long (at least 3 or 4 years) since I had last weighed myself that I had no idea what that number might be. I wondered how I would react to the question, and whether or not I would step on that scale.

Rather than getting stressed out, I decided to treat this situation as an experiment and observe my feelings and reactions. When the nurse asked me to step on the scale, I was surprised by my initial reaction—fear. What if I step on it and like the number? What if I don't like the number? What if this puts me back on the treadmill of up-and-down weight shifting. Would I be weighing my self-esteem again? It only took me a second to make the decision. I had to know—not the number, but whether I was still fixated with the weight.

So I took a deep breath and stepped on. I watched as the nurse slid the bar up and noted that the kilograms meant nothing. I waited for the nurse to translate it into pounds. When she told me the number, I wanted to laugh! Feelings of amazement and joy and freedom went swirling around my head! It was a non-number! It meant nothing! Zip! I can't even remember what it was! I had nothing to compare it to. I was truly free from the weight of that dreaded scale. I could be me. Me and my non-number—confirmation that I am definitely looking beyond my size to who I truly am.

As Christie has learned, once you've made the leap to the diet-free lifestyle, the tyranny of the scales can be broken. The sense of freedom it gives is incredible. When you've got a health-care provider that respects and understands how important this is, that's great. But sometimes doctors are just too wedded to their old ways of thinking. See what Carol Johnson has to say about that!

HERSTORY

Standing Up for Your Rights, *by Carol Johnson*

We've all heard it at one time or another—a doctor's brusque admonition "Your problem is you need to lose weight!" And most of the time we sheepishly agreed, not knowing what else to say. But when the weight doesn't come off, or when we lose weight only to regain it, we're afraid to go back to face the doctor.

This is what's happening among far too many larger people—they're simply avoiding their doctors, in fear of receiving "the lecture." I have long contended that if larger people do indeed have more health problems, in many cases it's not because they're fat, but because they aren't going in for preventative care.

People of the larger persuasion (and I am one) have the same right to medical care that a thin person has. And it's time we started asserting that right. We tend to forget that we are the customers, and we deserve to be treated with respect, understanding, and sensitivity. But it's time for a change!

I once had an internist who prescribed weight loss to cure whatever ailed me. He was nice enough about it, and so was I when I replied: "I've been trying to get thin my whole life, and it doesn't appear to be in the cards for me. I don't and won't diet. In the long run, it's probably made me fatter. So now I'm just trying to be healthy. I eat in a healthy manner the majority of the time, and I exercise regularly. I'm doing the best I can." His response: "Then that's all I can ask of you." Our relationship was just fine from that point on. He never prescribed a weight-loss diet, and I accepted responsibility for doing all that I could to develop a healthy lifestyle.

But keep in mind that medical problems are not confined to larger people. Lots of thin people have high blood pressure. Two of the thinnest people I know have severe back problems. I don't deny that there may be some conditions, such as Type II diabetes, that seem to be prevalent in larger people, but recently there's been a "chicken-or-egg" debate occurring as to whether obesity leads to diabetes, or diabetes promotes the development of obesity.

So what can you do when you're faced with "the lecture?" You don't have to argue. You can say something like this: "Yes, losing weight might help, but despite my best efforts, I haven't been able to do that. Over the long run, dieting has actually caused me to gain more weight. I don't want to continue in that pattern. So I now prefer to concentrate on improving my overall health, and I'll be glad to discuss ways of doing that. It may not be possible to be thin, but I can try to be healthy."

If, as I do, you keep up with the research of obesity, you can also say, "Researchers pretty much agree that we don't have a permanent cure for obesity yet, but a recent study showed that larger people who exercise regularly were quite healthy."

So how do you find a size-friendly doctor? You ask around. In my nondiet support group, "Largely Positive," we have developed a "size-friendly doctor list." Whenever one of our members has a pleasant experience with a doctor, we add that name to our list.

You can also do what another Largely Positive member did—you can interview prospective doctors. One member wrote a letter to her prospective doctor, explaining that she was a large woman and asking if that would present any problems for him. He had his assistant call back to say no, it wouldn't. You could also do this by telephone, but the letter approach allows the doctor to read your inquiry at his or her leisure—and it lets you have your say without interruption.

Some other things to keep in mind when facing a visit to the doctor:

- You don't have to be weighed unless there is a specific medical purpose, such as an impending operation requiring anesthesia. I just say nicely, "I don't care to be weighed," and I've never had a problem.

- If the gowns are too small, say so! The first time I visited my gynecologist and he gave me a paper sheet, I felt like I was trying to wrap a napkin around me. I told him next time I'd bring my own sheet and I did. He was sure surprised when I walked in and he saw me in a flowered bed sheet. He now has larger examination sheets!

- If your arm is very large, ask to have your blood pressure taken with a large sized-cuff. It can make quite a difference. When I asked my internist to do this he said, "But your arm isn't really that big." I asked him to do it anyway, just to see. My blood pressure was down almost 20 points with the larger cuff. My doctor's reply: "You've made a believer out of me!"

The bottom line is that you are entitled to the same medical care that a thin person would receive. Just telling a person with high blood pressure to lose weight is not acceptable treatment. You must demand the same treatment that a thin person would receive.

I don't mean to lambaste the entire medical profession. I have encountered many doctors who support our "largely positive" approach to health. So now go out and find one of them!

Remember, communication with your doctor is essential. You have every right to insist that your health-care provider respect your wishes about living a diet-free lifestyle, but you can't get that respect if you don't talk about it. And sometimes the doctor may think he has a specific reason for suggesting a weight reduction program —again, you won't know unless you ask. Here are a few words of wisdom from Penny on the subject.

So *That's* Why He Wants Me to Lose Weight, *By Penny Muir*

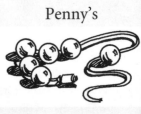

Penny's

Pearls

My friend and I have the same doctor. She and I went through the HUGS 10-week program together. I have worked through HUGS and noticed some change in my size and a tremendous change in my attitude. I am living life, feeling terrific and confident. My friend on the other hand, has continued in the diet mentality, despite my attempts to help her see the nondiet light. Her weight has increased (mind you, she has had a second baby) and she feels awful about it.

We both recently had appointments with the doctor. After her appointment, my friend told me that the doctor was very concerned about her weight, that she needed to work harder on losing the weight, and that the doctor was arranging for her to see a dietitian to get some nutrition counseling.

I saw the doctor that very same week regarding some asthma trouble I had recently been having. I suggested to him that some of my breathing difficulty may be due to inactivity and weight. I continued by saying that I'm kind of caught at the moment because my breathing difficulty makes it harder for me to exercise. I also took the time to mention that obesity is a family trait and I was concerned about fighting it.

My doctor told me that he has NO concern about me and my weight and that my breathing difficulty is a chronic disorder that requires constant monitoring but was unrelated to my weight. He said he was concerned about my husband's weight because there is a direct correlation between his weight and his (high) blood pressure but that in my case, my weight is *not* a health issue. He went on to tell me that with a slight change in my husband's lifestyle—fewer fast-food lunches and some stress reducing exercise—things would drastically improve. I spoke with my friend some more about her visit to the doctor and she told me that her blood pressure is way up, she is borderline diabetic, and she gets winded easily.

To my friend, our doctor seems to be one of those diet-focused doctors. To me, he is very enlightened in the nondiet way. I am glad I had the discussion with him about my health and weight concerns. The point: Communication (even when it looks like arguing) with your doctor is very important. Find out *exactly* why a doctor or health-care professional is stressing weight loss. If it is a matter of a health care professional being stuck in the diet mentality, then a change of doctors may be needed. But if your doctor raises real underlying health problems, then be sure to initiate a true dialogue, so that both you and your health-care professional clearly understand each other's concerns. Current research shows that your mutual health goals can most likely be achieved *without* resorting to a focus on weight loss! Stephen Blair, M.D. at the Cooper Institute in Texas has published extensive data showing that people can reduce their risk of chronic disease and improve their blood pressure, blood sugar, and cholesterol levels by becoming more physically active regardless of whether or not they lose weight.

Taking It Deeper

- **On: What's Up Doc?**

  1. The media bombards us daily with the words "health," "healthy lifestyle," "wellness," and "lean living." What do they actually mean? The media sends us many messages about what it means to be healthy. From all the mixed messages who and what do we believe?

     In this chapter you've been given the word power to arm yourself against the "diet talk" of health professionals. Get a buddy to role-play a scenario in which he or she is the doctor and you are the client. Practice it so that it becomes second nature.

- **On: Converting my Doctor**

  1. Have you had a trip to the doctor like Heather's, in which you successfully explained your nondiet lifestyle? If not, review the way that she handled the situation and see if her dialogue with her doctor has insights that you can use.

  2. "I'm not losing weight so my doctor says that the program is not working for me." How would you respond to such a comment from your doctor or health professional?

- **On: Me and My Non-Number**

  1. Discuss Mary's rear view approach to the scale in the doctor's office.

  2. What was Christie's approach? Discuss. How did taking action free them from the bonds of the scale? Have you tried this out? Try role-playing a similar scenario with a friend.

- **On: Standing Up for Your Rights**

  1. What phrases do you use when you encounter size prejudice from health professionals?

  2. Discuss your positive and negative experiences with the medical profession.

  3. Note and discuss the helpful ideas in Carol's article about how to turn around those negative experiences.

- **On: So *That's* Why He Wants Me to Lose Weight**

  1. Examine your relationship with your doctor or health-care professional. Are you comfortable questioning his or her advice to you? If not, why not?

  2. If you need to discuss diet and health related advice your doctor has given you, book a consultation appointment just to talk. Most good practitioners will accommodate an open, non-hurried discussion. If yours won't, consider re-evaluating your relationship and perhaps making a change.

Support Yourself

5

You Can't *Really* Live Without It
Seeking Support
Become Your Own Best Friend
How's *Your* Support Network?
Constructive Criticism Counts, Too
How Support Can Change Lives
Learning from the World of Nature

"Two are better than one, because they have a good reward for their toil. For if they fall, one will lift up the other; but woe to those who are alone when they fall and have not another to lift them up." (*Ecclesiastes* 4:9–10)

I f you were ever the butt of a schoolyard fat joke, then you know how early in life prejudice against overweight people begins. Being at the receiving end of this prejudice can lead to a lifetime of social isolation. The result: the very skills needed to interact socially are poorly—or never—developed. Cultivating friendships is an ongoing activity, but low self-esteem and lack of self-confidence makes that effort seem overwhelming.

For someone who wants to break away from the all-pervasive prejudice against "living large," however, a social network can be a lifesaver. You'd be amazed at how much easier it is to make changes in your lifestyle when you've got the support of one or more friends or acquaintances. While developing my HUGS program, I ran across a very helpful chapter on social support in a book by John P. Foreyt and G. Ken Goodrick, entitled *Living Without Dieting* (Warner Books, 1994). I have incorporated many of their insights on the value of a social support system into my own philosophy of a diet-free lifestyle, and offer them to you here, in this chapter.

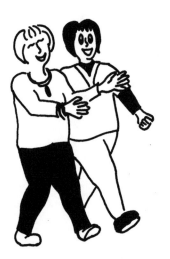

You Can't *Really* Live Without It

Some people avoid seeking support because they are uncomfortable in groups. But I would argue that if this is true for you, that's all the more reason to join one. Your resistance is probably due to feelings of insecurity, fears that you won't be accepted. But consider this: Joining a support group might *sound* scary, but support groups—by their very nature—*are* accepting.

There's another reason to find a support group—it improves the quality of your life immensely. It's no exaggeration to say that only through relating to and connecting with others will you achieve true happiness and fulfillment. You simply can't live a completely fulfilling life when you're socially isolated. And don't worry about being awkward at first: you'll get "good" at belonging to a group much more quickly than you think.

There are lots of benefits that come from developing a social support system—whether it's through a structured support group or through your own network of friends or family. According to Foreyt and Goodrick, a well-developed support system:

- Boosts self-esteem
- Brings in people who can offer good advice
- Validates your feelings, thus helping you to feel accepted and normal
- Boosts your success at making important changes in your lifestyle or other endeavors
- Helps you avoid over- and under-eating by giving you people to turn to when temptation arises
- Enriches your life by surrounding you with people with whom you can share experiences and even affection
- Helps you realize that you are valuable
- Helps you through crises
- Offers encouragement, so you can attempt things you've always wanted
- Lets you share emotions
- Confronts you with the truth, making it possible to break free of destructive patterns
- Offers valuable feedback

Seeking Support

It used to be that most of us could rely on our families for support, but things have changed during the last half of the twentieth century. As people became more mobile and independent, the nuclear family has replaced the extended family structure of previous generations. And as the nuclear family became the norm, it may even have begun to propagate destructive lessons. For example, many over-extended parents seem to have become under-involved with the eating habits and appearance of their children. Under-involvement can result in children fending for themselves, making

> Support comes in many forms. You can enlist a support buddy, join a local or online support group, start keeping a journal, read self-help books, listen to affirming audiotapes, or even hire a personal trainer!
>
> With all these options, surely there's a support system out there that's right for *you*!

inappropriate food choices that eventually become ingrained, setting up a lifetime of poor nutritional habits.

Alternatively, some parents have become over-involved in these same areas of their children's lives, obsessing about their children's weight. But such over-involvement often leads to the development of eating disorders and other psychological problems relating to food. If you grew up in either of these two circumstances, you may find it particularly difficult to switch to a nondiet approach on your own. That's why support systems are so important.

Become Your Own Best Friend, *By Penny Muir*

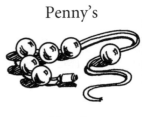

Penny's

Pearls

Talking to yourself by keeping a journal is a great form of support, so long as you build in positive feedback throughout the process. When I'm feeling vulnerable and a little out of touch, I find that it helps to write those feelings in my journal and then read them back to myself a little later. When I do this, I can see where I was feeling a little vulnerable, maybe a bit unreasonable, or where I was being kind of hard on myself. When dealing with myself and my own feelings, I need to look back on my words and feelings and say, "If those were the words of my friend, what would I say to encourage her?" I have learned through this process that I am my own best friend first. Support can come in many forms, and when outside support isn't there, learn to be your own best friend instead of your own worst enemy.

How's *Your* Support Network?

Assess the strength and variety in your support network right now. How many of the various types of support do you have available to you? If you are in a circle where you are only getting limited kinds of support, you are not going to grow, so be analytical about the support you get from each of your support sources, including the support provided by your friends or relatives.

For example, let's say that you can count on your sister, Sally, to hit you with the hard truth—even when that truth could be hurtful. Her "support," then, may erode some of your confidence—which can affect your self-esteem. Your friend Jane, on the other hand, may offer encouragement—and *boost* your self-esteem. Cousin Andrea may be great at helping you through a crisis and at offering helpful advice, while your co-worker, Sara, may have experienced a similar situation to one you're coping with, so she can share your experience and identify with your emotions. The idea is to become aware of the type of support you receive from each of your friends and acquaintances, so that when you need a shoulder to lean on you can turn to the person—or people—who can provide the most appropriate (and constructive) feedback.

When you review the many benefits that support provides, from improving your self-esteem to providing support during crises and supplying you with feedback on how well you're doing in an endeavor, you can easily see how unlikely—even unfair —it would be to expect that just one person could shoulder all that responsibility. That's why it is far better to have several friends to call on to provide support in one or more of these areas. After all, if you are getting self-esteem boosts, that's great—but boosts in self-esteem without helpful advice, or encouragement without feedback and validation, means that your system, however helpful, is still incomplete.

Constructive Criticism Counts, Too

The mature person comes to realize that receiving support means more than simply getting a pat on the back or other feel-good treatment—sometimes the best support is when a friend is willing to help you face a hard truth. And when you're trying to do something as life-changing as getting off—and staying off—the diet rollercoaster, you'll really need a lot of ongoing support to confront all the negative, pro-dieting messages that bombard you, such as unrealistic, idealized body types and ways of eating. That's why it's so very important to build a strong, well-balanced support system.

I recently got the opportunity to experience the full range of my own support network while writing the revised edition of my first book, *You Count, Calories Don't*. I was pleased that I could clearly see how drawing on the strengths of others had helped me bring the process all together. Each of my supportive friends offered me their unique skills and perspectives to help me in my work, and without their help I know my task would have been far more difficult, and far less rewarding.

- **Heidi**—generous and flexible—has shown me how to see things as a whole, to make everyday moments special, and to create memories.
- **Karen**—a patient, systematic planner—has been an inspiration with her entrepreneurial spirit, strong family values, practicality, and creativity.
- **Sandra**—insightful analyzer and good listener—shares laughs and tribulations with me, and we serve as mentors to each other. Each month we build in a special time during which we go out for a nice, long dinner and

talk things out. We come back rejuvenated, inspired, and grateful for each other's support.

- **Val**—wise, courageous, and full of integrity—has become my spiritual coach and is helping me on my journey to connect with and experience my own spirituality. She has helped me to understand how to grow in this manner. Her wisdom has guided me in learning to appreciate what I have—and how to enjoy the path I am taking.

- **Vicki**—persevering, conserving—she guides me in everyday living and inspires me with demonstrations of how to take the everyday gifts of nature around us and make them into something very special—from creating decorative arrangements of fallen leaves to weaving a tapestry inspired by the clouds in a blue sky.

These strong, creative, resourceful women have helped me to grow gracefully, and they've helped me make—and sustain—important changes in my life. It is equally important for you to develop and nurture a support system of your own—whether you draw upon your circle of friends and family, or join a group dedicated to providing this type of assistance.

How Support Can Change Lives

My experience has been that changes cannot be sustained unless support is built into your thinking right off the bat. Reading and self-reflection can stimulate your motivation to change, and can also bring more support in your life if you need it —they, too, are an important part of your support system. Books, especially, can provide invaluable support. For example, you can use this book for support by putting yourself in the personal situations shared by others who are working for change just as you are, and claiming the growth they have earned for your own.

Here are just a few more of those personal stories—this time, tales of how sharing and support have helped real people make real changes. The stories come from several women who formed a support group formed after they had completed a HUGS program session, so the concepts to which they refer are largely drawn from the HUGS program. Use their experience to encourage and inspire you in forming your own support group.

Kathy DeBacker: This support group has been a lifeline. To be able to share and talk about my joys, my progress, my pain and frustration, and life in general has been essential for me. The group has been a haven of acceptance, guidance, and support.

The HUGS course has actually become more important and useful to me in the months after the course than it was during the short eight weeks of the class. I am now able to understand and apply the principles of the program more effectively. I think in the beginning I was trying too hard and wanting the famous "instant results." The program has taught me self-acceptance, to savor each step of the journey, and most importantly patience. It was wonderful to find out that there really is no specific destination—just the wonderful, sometimes very painful process of evolving and changing, going forward and sometimes taking a step back.

Heather (the facilitator) has been an "angel" of wisdom, humor, and acceptance. I have learned so much from her and the journey she is on for herself. The other women have been so wonderful and supportive. They have taught me so much. I love them and the time we spend together.

Amber Bessant: I have really enjoyed coming to this program. It has taught me that I should accept myself the way I am. Before I joined, I really didn't like myself. Now I don't notice such negative things. Being in this group is absolutely wonderful because of the other people here. They can relate to how you are feeling and this can be truly beneficial.

Arlene Patterson: When I first heard of HUGS I wondered what the letters meant. Now that I have been in the group I have invented my own meaning for the letters: Human Understanding through Group Support. The group support is the best part! Getting together and talking it out has meant the most to me. I really look forward to the session. It is like a little boost that keeps you going with some new ideas to think about each time. One of the most amazing things about the support group has been the new perspectives and ways of looking at things that I never thought of before.

Brenda Peters: This support group has encouraged me to love who I am right now. One week at the support group we were all supposed to wear something that we wouldn't normally go out in public in. I had a dress on that I never wear because I always thought it was too tight and too short. I wore it to our support group and got so many compliments on it that I decided to be brave and wear it to church. I think I was testing to see if the support group were being honest with their compliments. Well, I've worn it twice and both times got favorable comments on it.

I really look forward to sharing my frustrations and also just reflecting over the past month. It really helps me to put things in perspective when I am able to articulate the struggles and victories I've had. For me journaling has been a positive thing. By writing thoughts and feelings down after I have eaten, I have realized why I have been putting food into my mouth when I've really needed to work through something else.

Heather Wiebe Hildebrand: When I think about the support group, it makes me smile. The group as a whole reminds me of myself. They seem to reflect a lot of my joys, challenges and struggles, and successes. I drive a little over an hour to get to the small town where it's held and I have to admit that sometimes I really dread the drive. However, each time we meet, I am so glad I came.

Some of the things that have really stuck out for me are:

- People who were filled with self-loathing are starting to like themselves the way they are.
- Some are journaling and gaining new insights into their patterns of emotions, attitudes, eating habits, and activity.
- Some have found out how much fun it is to be active and how good their body and mind feels during and after movement.
- Some have had the courage to wear beautiful trendy clothes and gone out dancing.

Each frustration and each success that is shared makes me feel that these group sessions are making a difference. The biggest joy for me in these support group meetings has been that beautiful people are finally discovering just how beautiful they are.

Learning from the World of Nature

An unexpected model of wisdom emerges from understanding the patterns of geese. Claim these lessons for your own situation. Describe specifically how you can take a small step to strengthen your personal network.

The Geese	The Lesson	Your notes on the lesson
As each bird flaps its wings, it creates an air draft for use by the bird following. By flying in a V formation, the whole flock adds 71 percent more flying range than if the bird flew alone.	People who share a common direction and sense of community can get where they are going more quickly and easily because they are traveling on the thrust of one another.	
Whenever a goose falls out of formation, it suddenly feels the drag and resistance of trying to fly alone, and quickly gets back into formation to take advantage of the lifting power of the bird immediately in front.	If we have as much sense as a goose, we will stay in formation with those who are headed where we want to go (and as we are willing to accept their help, we will also be willing to give our help to others).	
When the lead goose gets tired, it rotates to the back of the formation and another goose flies at the point position.	It pays to take turns doing the hard tasks and sharing leadership—with people, as with geese, we are interdependent on each other.	
The geese in formation honk from behind to encourage those up front to keep up their speed.	We need to make sure our honking from behind is encouraging—and not something else.	
When a goose gets sick or wounded or is shot down, two geese drop out of the formation and follow it down to help and protect it. They stay with it until it is able to fly again, or dies. Then they launch out on their own, with another formation, or catch up with their original flock.	If we have as much sense as geese, we too will stand by each other in difficult times as well as when we are strong.	

Taking It Deeper

- **On: You Can't Really Live Without It**

  1. Go back to the support-benefits list at the start of the chapter. Think about the people you know that can be relied upon to provide each of these types of support. Assess the particular skills and abilities each of these people have, and match up their names with the type of support they're each best at providing. Their support will be key in helping you to learn, grow, and stay with living a lifestyle without diets.

  2. Think about the kinds of groups you have been involved with in the past. Describe the rewards you received from this involvement.

  3. Examine how some past group experiences did not help you—and pay special attention to unsuccessful experiences with diet groups if you've belonged to those in the past. Assess what may have contributed to the failure of such group experiences—was it a lack of trust or courage on your part? An inappropriate group leadership style? Some other reason? If you can identify why previous experiences were not positive, you'll have a better chance at finding or creating a more positive group this time around.

- **On: Seeking Support**

  1. Reflect on the kind of social support your family provided when you were a child. Know that a mixture of good and bad aspects is normal. Do you think your parents had a particularly good or bad influence on your self-esteem and problems around eating?

  2. Do you believe that you are worthwhile enough to receive ample social support? If you feel unworthy, or are afraid that you wouldn't "belong" in a group, it's even more important to participate in order to have a better opinion of yourself. Try making a list of what you can bring to a support group—experiences you could share, sympathy and understanding you can provide—and you may feel more confident about being accepted.

- **On: Become Your Own Best Friend**

  1. Identify times when you were your own worst enemy and when you have been your own best friend.

  2. Examine your negative thoughts, vulnerable feelings, and life stresses. If your best friend turned to you for support on these things, what would you say to encourage her through a difficult time? Say—or write—those things to yourself.

  3. Don't forget your positive affirmations. Those positive thoughts running through your mind can be just the lift you need when you feel overwhelmed or vulnerable.

- **On: How Support Can Change Lives**

  1. Connect with a group of friends that want to give up dieting and look at an alternative. Carve out a specific weekly time period to get together and learn how to free yourselves from dieting. Feel free to use this book as a starting point to lead your own support group—you can use the "Taking It Deeper" sections as a source of discussion topics and activities. For additional support, go to www.hugs.com.

- **On: Learning from the World of Nature**

  1. Consider the insights available from the study of geese provided in the chart in this chapter. What lessons can you take from their example? Share your discoveries with a friend or your support group.

Resetting Your Stress Barometer

6

Getting Back into Balance
    Juggling home and work
    Keeping it real
I Count
Get Some Help
Virtual Support Groups
Get Busy Getting Not So Busy
    Getting a busy signal
    Getting rid of the guilts
Stop Taking Shortcuts to Stress
Slow Down the Vacation Rush
Combat Stress with Pen Power
Journaling

Stress can make you fat. All the chocolate, cookies, cakes, chips, and other stress foods you nibble on to temporarily quell the stress also put on the pounds. And when you're stressed, your willingness to exercise drops off, as do those vegetable-filled, healthy meals you were making for yourself—healthy habits are often the first thing to go when you're very busy and stressed out.

And stress may wear down another healthy resolve: to stop dieting—after all, it's hard enough to cope with a high-stress life without adding the difficulty of "swimming against the tide" of pro-diet thinking. But, as you know from the early chapters of this book, dieting can make you fat. To stay off the diet rollercoaster—and to enhance your life in a hundred other ways—it's therefore vital that you lower your stress level.

So take a minute to answer this question: Is your stress barometer permanently set on "high"? Part of staying energized is keeping the stress level somewhere in the middle range—a comfort zone where you are neither "rusting out" from under-stimulation nor "burning out" from over-stimulation. There are hundreds of books out there that you can turn to for advice on combating stress, so I won't try to give you the definitive approach in this chapter. Instead, I'll show you how stress relates to dieting, health, and other themes of this book. You'll get useful advice on lowering your stress barometer from me and other women committed to diet-free lifestyles. At the end of this chapter you'll receive a wonderful de-stressing tool: a simple journal.

Getting Back into Balance

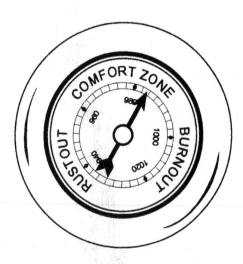

A huge source of stress is a lifestyle that has gone out of balance. Overworking, overeating, overdrinking, smoking, taking no time to yourself, devoting too much time to others, giving up on exercise . . . there are so *many* ways to lose balance.

Achieving balance in the first place is no easy task, especially if you're juggling career and family. And sometimes the "experts" are no help at all. Kim, a HUGS colleague of mine, once told me of a seminar she had attended on putting balance into her life. It was specifically addressed to working women with careers outside the home. But instead of helping them come up with creative ways of balancing home and career, the seminar's message was "either devote yourself to your career, or stay at home." There's that old, familiar all-or-nothing approach that we're trying to move beyond! As far as Kim was concerned, these seminar leaders were missing the point: the all–or–nothing way is what knocks our lives out of balance in the *first* place.

Juggling home and work

When stress is building up in your life, it's time to pull back and reassess what is *really* important to you. Most people realize that the special moments in life cannot be bought with money—yet the pursuit of money is a major "unbalancer" for a great many people. Juggling the demands of home and work can sometimes be too much to handle.

Many people resolve the work-versus-home conflict by working part-time, which allows them to spend an equivalent amount of family time as a means of achieving empowerment and balance. And some choose slightly less lucrative careers that offer the freedom to express themselves while achieving at least a minimum of financial independence, and the luxury of enjoying time with their family. Of course, not everyone has these options—but if stress is getting you down and you have the good fortune of having the skills or education that allow you to pull back from the conventional working world, by all means consider making a change. The part-time or self-employed person may have the best of both worlds. Balance in one's life is a fringe benefit that no full-time venture can offer.

In order to balance our lives, we need to feel that we have a choice. Feeling trapped? Broaden your mind a little, and you'll realize that yes, in fact, you do have choices. Stop and reflect on whether you're working your butt off for things that are *truly* important to you, or if you're slaving away to get something that, in the end, is less satisfying than spending some "special" time in front of the fire playing charades and laughing. Our fast-paced lifestyle is sometimes self-imposed, driven by our desire to have everything. Taking a "time out" to just be yourself can actually increase your efficiency when there is work to be done.

And if you choose to work full time because you do still need some material things that only money can buy, consider approaching your employer about flexible hours. For example, a work day that runs from noon to 8 p.m. can be very convenient. Such a schedule would give you some time during the morning hours in which you could relax and spend some time with your spouse before he (or she) heads off to work, and you'd have a chance to get at those daytime errands that everyone else has to rush to get done on their lunch hour or at quitting time. Moms with school-age kids could ask for a "split" work day—working while the kids are in school but heading home for a couple of hours when they're due back from school. Creative scheduling allows you to build into your life some precious moments. Why put such pleasures on hold until vacation time or retirement if you don't have to?

Keeping It Real

Unrealistic expectations of yourself are another sure way to throw you out of balance. We all are prone to thinking we have to be "super woman"—keeping a tidy home, raising the kids, and handling the demands of a job all at the same time. But those are three full-time jobs right there! Fight off these false expectations that you can and should ride out all problems with Amazon strength, never giving in to overwhelming emotions. Sometimes you've just got to let down that brave face and admit that you're feeling a little—okay, maybe a *lot*—overwhelmed.

There's a fine balance to strive for. Handling the problems of daily life is a worthy struggle. But for your own sake it's good to realize that you can't always put a brave face on things that happen—nor should you. After all, if you don't allow yourself to experience the "downs" of life every once in awhile, the "ups" won't really mean much. But honestly allowing yourself to experience the ups and downs of life doesn't mean giving yourself permission to exist in a perpetual mope, either—you want to face life with optimism, but be gentle with yourself on those occasions when the going temporarily gets to be too tough to take with a smile.

I Count, *by Christie Keating*

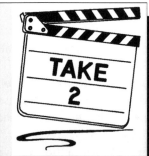

As a single parent, I am keenly aware of the lack of "me" time. So, recently, I decided to set aside some time, every day, for me. Selfish? No way!

Parents with partners can usually find a compromise to give each other time off. A give-and-take sort of arrangement. Single parents, unless there is a lot of support from family and friends, usually find their time off only after the kids are in bed and all the domestic duties are done. But by then, our beds look pretty appealing and I don't believe that time off necessarily includes sleeping.

It is my hope that my children will learn to appreciate that not only do I care for them, I also care for myself. I hope that this will instill in them the fact that the world does not revolve just around them, and that other members of the family (me) are just as important as they are. If I don't nurture and care for myself, I am sending them the message that I don't count. And I do. Here are my tricks for getting some "me" time—they may work for you, too:

- *Only 15 minutes:* By setting my alarm 15 minutes earlier, I will be able to enjoy padding through a quiet house to have my shower without listening for the kids' toast to pop.

- *I'm not the maid:* Yes, laundry still needs to be done, but hey, if the kids don't put it in the basket, too bad.

- *My turn:* The kids have play time; I want mine (and not after 11 p.m.). I will exercise my right to have my turn on the computer, or to sit quietly reading (uninterrupted), or even (bliss!) close my eyes for 20 minutes and listen to my favorite Celtic ballads.

- *I'm tired:* This is a perfectly OK statement to use if I really *am* tired! This goes hand in hand with "I can't listen intently right now, can you tell me a little later when I will have the energy to hear everything you're saying?"

- *My time:* Sometimes I give myself an extra splurge of indulgence. Making meals only *I* like. Messing my own house with my own mess. Staying up really late to take advantage of my time. Not using the time for housework. Eating in bed. Taking hikes that the kids say are too long. Playing my music as loud as I want!

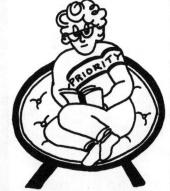

- *Rest the guilt:* This is the hardest one, the one that requires the most work. Taking time for me is not selfish. It is helping me to keep my sanity for one of life's most difficult and rewarding full-time jobs, parenthood.

Get Some Help

One thing I highly recommend when your life is over-stressed and out of balance is to turn to a support group network. Sure, they're there to support you in your quest to live a lifestyle without diets, but they can also help you put life back in balance. Because the members face

If there are no support groups conveniently located near you, try an online group. Newcomers are always welcome at the HUGS website: www.hugs.com

many of the same issues and pressures that you do, they can provide the camaraderie and inspiration that you need to deal with everyday problems or "blue-funk" depressions when you feel you're carrying too much. And while they're helping you cope with stress, they're supporting your efforts to face down society's diet- and size-hype!

Virtual Support Groups, *by Penny Muir*

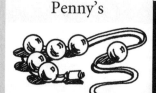

Penny's

Pearls

Internet chat rooms serve a positive purpose for many of us. Some use chat rooms or chat programs to converse with loved ones and save the long-distance phone charges. For many of us, however, these chat rooms and programs serve another purpose. They are virtual meeting rooms where we meet to discuss a range of topics and issues including everything from crafts and hobbies to parenting and just about anything that can be discussed in an open forum. Even HUGS has its own chat room.

I have participated in a number of virtual round-table discussions, mostly regarding parenting issues. I have met a number of wonderful parents from all corners of the world. We have shared the joys and the sorrows of parenting and step-parenting. There are special chats for parents of children of all age groups, chats for bereaved parents, and general chats where we can have grown-up discussions after a long day with the kids. These chats, together with my participation in the HUGS program, have prepared me to host my first scheduled chat at the HUGS website.

These chat room support networks succeed because they're there when the participant needs them. They fit into any busy schedule. There is no set time to be there to find someone that needs or can give support. The faceless person on the other end has real feelings but the anonymity of the computer allows feelings and ideas to flow between virtual strangers without difficulty.

Oftentimes when I log into the HUGS chat room there is someone else there who, like me, is trying to stay away from the kitchen or the scale. Many times I logged into the chat room because I felt out of control or lacking in strength. Invariably, I found someone else there struggling with a similar issue. Occasionally, I found someone there who was not struggling but was ready, willing, and able to remind me to analyze my thoughts, to read the pertinent literature to combat my struggle, to listen to my body signals, or to simply distract me long enough for my strength to return.

Acquiring good problem-solving skills helps cut back on stress. A lot of them are based on simple mnemonics—simple words or phrases that help you memorize the steps you can take to cut problems down to size. Two that I find particularly helpful are "PAST" and "Why not?" Here's how they work:

PAST

P   Identify your **PROBLEM**. Remember that most problems are really a series of small problems, not just one big one.

A   List your **ALTERNATIVES**. Be as free as you can in coming up with potential solutions.

S   Make your **SELECTION** of the best alternative in your list. You'll identify the best one by looking at the pros and cons in each one.

T   Give your solution a **TRYOUT**. If the alternative you selected didn't do the trick, go back to the list and find another one to try.

The "So What?" technique is even easier to try. All it takes is that you ask yourself three questions, whenever a problem threatens to overwhelm you:

So what is the problem?

So what can I do about it?

So what are the consequences of doing that?

Yes, the phrase "So What?" can drive you crazy when your kids overdo it, but it's actually a very useful approach to critical thinking and creative problem solving. Try it yourself. It's particularly recommended for those times when you recognize that you've become trapped in a situation that may be a barrier to moving on in your thinking or action and need a good self-talk session to get yourself jump-started again.

Get Busy Getting Not So Busy

How familiar does this exchange sound?

"So, how are you?"

"Busy," "I'm keeping busy," "Too busy right now"

These responses are common in everyday conversations. Indeed, the state of "busyness" is usually recognized as an admirable quality or positive attribute. But what kind of impact does this rushed lifestyle have on our health? Do we listen to our bodies for signs that it needs to pull back? Do we recognize that taking a rest or saying "no" to one more task is not evidence of a weakness in character?

Wondering if *you've* been overdoing it lately? Look for these signs:

- an inability to concentrate and focus
- always feeling fatigued
- feeling rushed
- feelings of anxiety or uneasiness
- feelings of irritability, impatience, or moodiness

This list is by no means exhaustive, however. Over time, each of us develops our personal symptoms that mean the pressure's rising on our personal stress barometers, and these symptoms can be very individualized. For example, one person may start neglecting household tasks that she normally takes in stride daily. Another person may start letting her personal hygiene slip. A third may stop preparing meals for herself, catching a quick (and not necessarily nutritious) bite on the run.

Getting a Busy Signal

Pay attention to your body's signals for rest and attention! Prolonged periods of ignoring them can lead to sickness down the road. We need to remember to be more gentle to ourselves and to take a break from the busyness of our lives. Are you taking time out when you need it?

Ask yourself: "When was the last time I pampered myself?" If the answer was longer than a week or so, ask yourself this: "What will happen to my health if I don't pay attention to my needs?" Now, here's the final question—the one that will get you back on the right track: "What new thing can I do for myself to build some 'time-outs' into my lifestyle?"

Think you don't have time to relax, that your schedule doesn't allow it? Then you're probably over-committed—you're doing too much giving and not enough receiving. This can be a sign that you're trying to please others in order to win their approval: a classic symptom of low self-esteem. To overcome this tendency, remember: This is *your* life and you have choices about how you want to live it. Taking time for yourself will reduce your stress level, put your life in balance, and enable you to put problem situations into better perspective.

Getting Rid of the Guilts

Our work-crazed culture can make you feel guilty taking time for yourself. But, as Penny Muir puts it: "I find when I don't take time for me, I'm irritable and short-tempered, and not as willing to give to others. When I take even 15 minutes a day just for me I am recharged, patient, and much more willing to give. Taking 'me' time isn't just something I deserve, it's something I need."

Feeling guilty won't allow you to enjoy the time spent alone or relaxing with your family. So remember, the time you spend on yourself will only come back to your family in your renewed happiness and sense of contentment. You deserve it. Learn to relax . . . and enjoy the moment.

Stop Taking Shortcuts To Stress

Saving time and saving money are the magic words in our fast-paced society. A headline about a shortcut grabs just as much attention as a headline about a freebie. It's only human nature to try to take shortcuts around the complex details of life but, ironically, shortcuts may only add to your stress.

We often carry the illusion that experts or more experienced folk have figured out easy ways to do things. Ask around when you have a project in mind and the advice you're apt to receive is that there *are* no shortcuts. What looks like a shortcut from the outside looking in is just smartly executed process!

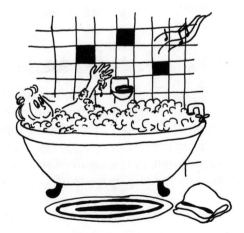

Of course, when you're faced with all the steps it takes to execute a project you can end up feeling as if you're buried in details. But even though the list of steps might look overwhelming, it actually puts you in control of the job. And as you finish each step, you have an achievement.

A Fence Painting Parable

We wanted to paint our fence. Our white rail fence, I must go on to tell you, surrounds our property of four-and-a-half acres, so this is no small undertaking. Here are the steps involved in the fence project.

1. Use weed eater to get rid of the weeds around the fence as they were as high as the fence.

2. Replace broken boards with new ones.

3. Scrape the fence to take off old paint.

4. Apply a primer coat to the fence boards.

5. And, finally, apply paint color.

What would happen if we tried to shortcut any of the steps? If we didn't get rid of the weeds around the fence it would be difficult and frustrating to get to the fence and actually paint it. If we didn't replace all the boards before we started painting, we'd have to do it as we went along, which means that the paintbrushes would dry out and the work would flow less efficiently. If we didn't scrape properly, the old paint would peel off and we'd be doing the job all over again in two years. And without the primer, the paint wouldn't adhere as well as it should.

Obviously, there's a reason for every step in the process. But we were only human —we tried a shortcut: we skipped the primer coat. We figured that since we scraped off the old paint we could get away without having to do this step. Result: We ended up using *so* much more of the expensive paint than we would have had to if we had primed the fence first. We saved some time, but were we actually further ahead?

OK, your turn: Reflect on a project that didn't quite work out the way it should and break it down into the steps you took to get it done. Note what you can do differently next time—what steps you may have skipped the first time around. This is the best way to learn from your setbacks—by allowing yourself to take a moment to reflect on what went wrong, you can usually find ways to do better next time. Most important is to learn to laugh at such setbacks. They're learning experiences, not failures!

If you apply this planning process to every aspect of life, you'll realize that there is a step-by step way to avoid most problems—or at least minimize them. In addition, when you break projects down into steps, you feel like you are moving forward, which gives you a sense of accomplishment and builds self-esteem. And since problems *do* occur even after careful planning, make sure to build in time to deal with them.

Slow Down the Vacation Rush

Vacations are often very stressful, even if you're normally cool and collected at other times during the year. Often we rush to get ready for vacation, push-push-push while we are there to get in all the "fun," and then rush back to plunk ourselves down into the work-a-day grind. Within days we're back to feeling like we never had a break at *all*! Well, if you treat your vacation like a project, you can make it different the next time.

On our recent vacation—a winter getaway to Orlando, Florida, with another family —I took a little time beforehand to break the trip down into three stages:

1. Planning the event

I started my planning well in advance, and talked about the upcoming vacation with friends and family to find out what they had done on similar trips. Anticipation became a part of the fun. We took everything bit by bit, so we weren't stuck packing and organizing in a mad rush at the last minute.

2. Experiencing the event

During the actual vacation, I tried to strike a balance between intense discovery time and time to relax and just hang out. That way we had time to absorb the experience. Without this balance, the day or even the week can become a fog. You forget the details—where you were and what you did. If you're traveling with friends, one good way to make the experience more "real" is to take on the role of "tour guide." My husband and I spend one full day covering a particular part of the park, and a few days later we went back there with the family we were vacationing with. The sights we had seen on our earlier visit became new because this time we saw them through someone else's eyes. We even saw things that we didn't notice the first time around.

3. Recapping the event

A vacation isn't necessarily over just because you've come home and now you've got to unpack and do the laundry. Part of any vacation is the reminiscing you can do: talking it up in interesting and entertaining anecdotes for your family and friends. This helps to cement the special time into your memory. When we got back from our vacation, my husband related some of our funny stories to his parents over a glass of sherry and I thought to myself: "Hmmm . . . that was really fun! We really *did* take in a lot of fun-filled events!" Replaying the events through stories, pictures, and mementos keeps the experience alive.

Using a process like this one can make any special time a part of your pleasant-memories bank. Try it out. Do you notice the difference? Think back on a former holiday and note what you could have done differently to make it that special memory that you desire, that you can call on at any time.

Combat Stress with Pen Power

A fabulous way to identify your sources of stress—and to assess your progress in the process of de-stressing—is to keep a journal. Putting aside some time with pen and paper can help you to work through the day's activities, appreciate the moment, and give you a focus for the day ahead. The process itself forces you to spend some time with yourself and helps you get to know yourself better. If nothing else, it interrupts the rush of your busy everyday daily activities and lets you focus on yourself instead of catering to the needs of others.

Keeping a journal—what we in HUGS call "journaling"—you have a chance to think, discuss, create, use the written word, and explore—all at once! In turn, you learn about chronicling, charting your progress, organizing, and venting in a positive way. Not everyone enjoys the written word, but everyone enjoys learning about themselves and what makes them tick, and then reading about it afterwards. What a great way to build self-esteem, confidence, and skills all at once! Whatever the reason, enjoy your decision to use pen power. Journaling is also a good opportunity to brag to yourself about your personal successes.

Journaling definitely puts you in touch with yourself and your feelings. Too often we bury our feelings deep down and only the superficial "you" is shown to others. Part of being a whole person means getting to understand that emotional part of you that has feelings of delight, anger, fear, frustration, anticipation, and the like. Sharing these feelings with others, or writing about them in your journal, will help you to understand them better. And your journal can provide you with a way to communicate with others, even when you're too shy to speak directly. Perhaps you know someone with whom you would like to confide—you can do so by sharing the contents of your personal journal. You could even exchange journals and discuss your individual discoveries and areas of growth. In the HUGS program, such a relationship is called "journal buddying."

As you keep up your journal, writing will become an automatic part of the day's activities—just like brushing your teeth. You may find it to be a very rewarding part of your day. Says HUGS graduate Penny Muir, "Journaling was very good for me. I was able to see patterns in my thinking, crisis management skills, and food choices. Things I wasn't able to see until I went back and re-read some of the entries. It really opened my eyes as to where I still indulged in diet thinking and where I was relying on food to fill the gaps."

Keep in mind that your journal is not the same thing as a diary. It's more than a mere record of the day's events. In your journal you explore your feelings about life's daily occurrences; you are candid about your reactions, and you explore changes you may make the next time similar events occur. The journal provides you with an opportunity to cherish precious moments and to revisit them whenever you choose to reread what you have written.

Here's what your journal does for you:

- It creates action: You can use the journal as a planning tool. When you write something down, you are more likely to turn your intentions into action, to actually carry them out.

- It builds responsibility: Writing about an issue in your journal is apt to instill a sense of responsibility—you are more likely to "own" your actions, emotions, or responses when you explore them in writing.

- It lets you chart your progress: From time to time you can look back through the entries in your journal and see how far you have come. If you don't detect progress, you can reflect on prior entries and try to discover what's stopping or blocking you.

If you've never kept a journal before, you may need a few tips on how to go about it. Here are some helpful ideas to get you started on your personal journal routine:

- Buy a book: Stationery departments stock lots of beautifully bound journals, some with blank pages, others complete with lined paper. Alternatively, you can pick up a loose leaf binder. Go with a fancy cover, or pick a plain one that you can customize. Spiral-bound notebooks, which come in a range of sizes, are also a good choice. If you're fully committed to the computer age, set up a file on your PC or laptop. The choices are as individual as you are.

- Making time: Because journaling is a personal experience, it's up to you to choose when to write. Some people set aside a particular time each day, others write whenever they feel like it. Keep in mind that there will be some days when you will have nothing to say—and that's OK. Journaling is a powerful tool that can help you work through personal issues, it is not a chore or a test.

- Can I Stop? While some people think journaling is so helpful that they keep it up throughout their lives, others see it solely as a way to organize and clarify their thoughts. In time you may discover that the thinking process that is nurtured by journaling has become automatic to you and you might choose to discontinue the writing. That's fine. It's up to you to decide how you want to use the process: as a stepping stone to achieving a balance in your life, as a way to linger with your thoughts, as a tool for working through problems, or as a special time for just you, alone.

HERSTORY

Journaling, *by Heather Todd*

I started writing in a journal when I was twelve. I have always used it as a way of recording the happiest, saddest, and most exciting events that have taken place and as a way of venting my feelings and thoughts. At the age of fourteen I developed an eating disorder and I began to write in my journal even more. I had a lot of negative emotions associated with the eating disorder, and I have found keeping a journal a good way to organize my thoughts and get out all the bad feelings instead of having them eat me up inside.

I have never set a definite schedule of when I have to write. I don't even write everyday. I just do it whenever the mood takes me. The only times that I will almost always write is after appointments with my doctor or psychologist, and after attending the eating disorder support group. This way I can keep track of what we discussed instead of just pushing it to the back of my mind. There may have been a really good idea or suggestion that I wasn't ready to use at the time and forgot about. Then if I read back at another time I may decide to use it.

When I read back in my journal I find it's a good way of seeing whether or not I am making progress in my recovery with the eating disorder. The only downside I have found is that I will sometimes write negative things about myself, or see that I am not making any progress in recovery and on re-reading such entries I tend to feel worse about myself. Overall though, I have found writing in a journal a very positive experience and strongly recommend it to others.

Taking It Deeper

- **On: Getting Back into Balance**

  1. If you're juggling a career and home life, try coming up with choices —no matter how small they are—that can reduce the demands that these two areas of life place upon you. Consider what you're working for, and what you truly want to achieve, and see where changes can be made.

  2. Discuss ways in which you can improve the balance between fulfilling your responsibilities and building in personal time for refreshment and renewal.

  3. Discuss the idea that difficult times provide us the opportunity to grow and strengthen our character and enrich our ability to appreciate the good times. Is it realistic to expect that we feel upbeat all the time?

- **On: I Count**

  1. Are Christie's "I Count" ideas workable in your life? Why was it important for Christie to build in time for herself? How can this help other members of her family?

  2. Look over Christie's ideas for "my time." What special activities would you add to such a list?

- **On: Get Some Help**

  1. Discuss how a support buddy or group can help you through hard times or give you a new perspective. Give examples of how allowing the sadness to surface and the natural grieving process to occur eventually can lead to acceptance.

- **On: Virtual Support Groups**

  1. Discuss how chat rooms and message boards offer a form of support.

2. Penny writes, "The faceless person on the other end has real feelings but the anonymity of the computer allows feelings and ideas to flow between virtual strangers without difficulty." Drop in for a visit at the HUGS Web site and visit our support group. If you're new to chat rooms, remember that you can just watch others as they participate, until you feel comfortable about jumping in.

- **On: Problem Solving**

1. Define a problem that you face with some frequency and try working it out using the PAST and "So What" problem solving techniques. If you're working through this section with a friend or a support group, take turns posing problems and responding to them.

- **On: Get Busy Getting Not So Busy**

1. Check your own stress barometer: Are you rusting out? Heading to burnout? Or safely within the comfort zone? Think back on high-stress periods of your life and give examples of what you did to restore your balance.

2. Consider how long ago was the last time you pampered yourself. Is it time to start building in some regular "time out" for yourself? What benefits can you expect to come from such "me" time?

- **On: Stop Taking Shortcuts to Stress**

1. Discuss the difference between getting a job done efficiently and taking a shortcut. Use the fence-painting story to illustrate your discussion.

2. Practice logically analyzing projects or tasks. Pick a job that needs doing and break it down into necessary steps. Using the steps as your guide, perform the job and see how much more control you have over the outcome.

- **On: Slow Down the Vacation Rush**

1. Discuss what you can do differently in planning your next vacation. Have you ever considered taking more frequent mini-holidays to re-energize instead of just going for the "let's save up those three

weeks and take them all at once" and then have to wait an entire year for the next break? Do you see some of that all-or-nothing thinking creeping in?

- **On: Combating Stress With Pen Power**

  1. Review Heather Todd's story about journaling. Discuss how she has used journaling to cope with problems. What are other ways that journaling might be useful to you?

  2. Try keeping a journal yourself. Give it a try for a few days, at first. Do you find that it helps you clarify your thoughts and feelings?

  3. If you are working through this book with a friend or participating in a support group, share your journal insights. Use journal entries as a starting point to discuss the process of changing to a lifestyle without diets.

88

A Self-Esteem Shot In the Arm 7

My Scale Moves Around but I Stay the Same
How's Your Self-Esteem?
    Who's in charge?
    How to score
    Ten steps to loving your body just as it is
Change That Tape in Your Head
Finding the Courage
My Body or My "Problem Areas"
Cleaning Out the Closet
Thin Clothes, Fat Clothes
Getting a Real Life
Stop Playing the Numbers
Riding High and Free

Among the many assaults society makes on our self-esteem, dieting has got to rank *way* up there. Linking your self-esteem to a number on the scale, as society tells us we should do, is terribly demoralizing. If you've been dieting on and off, you know the drill: your weight goes down, you feel good; as it goes up, you feel awful. On weigh-in day at the doctors office or the diet group, you don't eat all day so that you'll be just a little bit lighter when you step on the scales . . . so that you'll feel a little bit successful, no matter how small the weight loss.

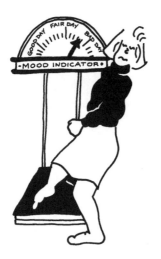

But this mentality and focus on weight as a measure of success not only discourages healthy eating habits, it also encourages starve-and-binge eating cycles, and it is devastating to your self-esteem. This chapter is about all sorts of ways to boost self-esteem—and one of the most important of these ways is to disconnect your sense of self-worth from your weight by basing your self-esteem on your own, unique, internal qualities.

In this chapter I'm letting Penny, Heather, and a few others tell most of the self-esteem tale. They share stories of how they came to accept themselves, how they learned to accept their bodies even when they don't conform to current Western standards of beauty, and how they regained joy and freedom in their lives. In their brave recollections, they offer many paths to developing self-esteem. I hope their stories will inspire you to build up your own sense of worth, or to reconstitute it when it begins drying up.

My Scale Moves Around, but I Stay the Same, *by Penny Muir*

Penny's

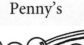

Pearls

Back in my dieting days I learned that even after my diet goal was achieved, I was still the very same person inside. The attention I received, and the self-esteem boost I felt when I lost weight were short-lived—as was the weight loss itself. Changing myself on the outside did little or nothing to change who I felt I really was inside, and so I quickly fell back to old habits of turning to food for all the things I thought I lacked. No wonder that the weight I lost (and more) always came back.

How's Your Self-Esteem?

Before we get too far into the self-esteem stories of our friends Penny, Heather, and a few others, why not take a minute to assess your own self-esteem. Here's a quiz that will give you a self-esteem "reading" right now. But, just like you're doing with the Diet Mentality Quiz that you first found in Chapter 1, it's a good idea to retake this quiz every once in a while. You'll be pleased to know that as you move further and further away from the diet mentality, your self-esteem score will more than likely increase.

Who's in charge?

One indicator of self-esteem is the amount of control you have—or feel that you have—over your life. Try this test, adapted and used with permission from The Best You Can Be Nutrition Program, Regional Public Health, David Thomas Health Region, Alberta, Canada.

Who's In Charge Of . . .	Me	Spouse	Both of us	Family	Circumstances	Colleagues
My hair color						
My hairstyle						
What I wear in public						
What I wear at home						
What I eat						
Where I eat						
What I do for physical activity						
How much exercise I get						
What I read						
What I watch on TV						
What music I listen to						
My bedtime						

If it's time to "make a change"						
How confident I feel						
How I decorate my home						
How I spend my free time						
How much time I spend with friends						
How much time I spend with family						
How I spend my solitary free time						
If I'm healthy						
The size of my household budget						
The size of my personal budget						
How I spend my personal budget						
What kind of job or career I have						
How many hours I spend on my job						
What I should weigh						
What I should eat						
TOTALS:						

How to score:

Each check in the "Me" box counts as one point. Checks in other boxes don't count at all. So add up all the checks in the "Me" box.

If your score is 25–27: Congratulations! You are totally in charge of your life and it feels good, doesn't it?

If your score is 20–24: You, too, have a handle on a balanced life in which you are generally comfortable with the decisions you make. Look at those areas where others may influence—or even make—your decisions for you. Ask yourself how you feel about this and whether or not you would like to change it.

If your score is 15–19: About half of your decisions are made by someone else. You may feel powerless to do what you really want. You may not even know what you really want, because others so frequently make your decisions for you. Re-examine the areas where you are *not* the decision maker and consider why this might be so. Talk it over with others to get some ideas on what you can do to take back some control over decision-making in your own life.

If your score is under 15: This is a warning sign. Your self-esteem may be so low that you are letting others tell you what to do and how to live your life. Ask yourself, "how does it feel when you actually make a decision." Would you like to do this more often? You may need some guidance to help you to become more assertive if you are unable to do it on your own—that's where getting support from friends, support groups, or family can be crucial to your success in making a change.

Ten steps to loving your body just as it is

The Council on Size and Weight Discrimination, Inc., has some great suggestions for learning to love yourself just the way you are. Here are their ten tips for improving your self-esteem:

1. Be around people who accept themselves as they are. Join a support group—or start one if necessary—and talk and listen to others who are on the same path.

2. Read books, pamphlets, and articles on self-acceptance; look at art; and watch films and videos with strong, beautiful characters of different sizes and shapes.

3. Buy full-length mirrors and appreciate yourself from all directions. Look at yourself standing, sitting, from the back, naked, clothed— every way.

4. Look your best. Buy and wear great clothes you like and feel good in. Get rid of uncomfortable and ill-fitting clothing, and anything you've been saving "until it fits." Getting a new hair style can do wonders.

5. Take pictures of yourself. Let others take pictures of you. Don't avoid being in group pictures—in fact, insist on standing in the front.

6. Stop being so hard on yourself.

7. Start acting as if you love—and have always loved—your body.

8. Learn to recognize size discrimination, diet obsession, fat phobia, and body hatred in the world around you—in advertising, in television and movies, in public accommodations, on the street, among your family and friends, and in your *own* thinking.

9. Start the process of "coming out" as a self-accepting person by telling your family, friends, co-workers, and others of your decision to stop obsessing about your weight and appearance, to give up dieting and the goal of losing weight, and to accept yourself and your looks as you are.

10. Become an advocate for the rights of people of any size, shape, color, ability, or physical appearance. Interrupt sizism, racism, lookism, ableism, sexism, and other prejudiced attitudes wherever you encounter them.

Change That Tape in Your Head (or Discoveries from a Soup Bowl), *by Heather Wiebe Hildebrand*

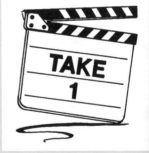

In order to make a good soup you have to start with a good soup stock. The base can make or break a good bowl of soup. Like soup's different flavors and textures, we are all different, but we can all be successful in achieving healthier lifestyles if we start with a good base. We may take different routes to success and use different styles, but there are a few basics that are universal.

Self-acceptance: One of the basics I discovered was that I actually had to learn how to like myself the way I was before moving on to other issues. Why was this so important? Well, because when I didn't like "Heather," I wasn't very effective in looking after her. I would eat whenever I was upset and blame others for it. I didn't listen to my body's signals of hunger and fullness. I practiced "all or nothing" thinking in my activities and eating patterns. When I didn't feel good about myself, I was filled with negative emotions and had less energy to be good to myself. I found I needed to focus on positive things and this created energy to make healthier choices in my life.

Change the inner dialogue: I tried saying, "I like myself the way I am," but my inner dialogue was, "RIGHT! How can I like myself the way I am? I am a lumpy, bumpy individual with more flaws than I care to identify." Changing that inner dialogue has probably been the most difficult lifestyle change to make. I was not a big fan of affirmation tapes, but I had to try something, anything, so I tried them. Daily I would repeat, "I like myself the way I am. I feel good about myself, I am going to have a great day." In the beginning I would say it and laugh. Some days I couldn't even say it. Other days I would say it and feel like crying. Some mornings the only reason I would affirm myself was because my husband would drag me to the mirror and make me say, "Heather, you like yourself the way you are."

Slowly but surely I started to believe what I was saying. I started to enjoy the way I looked in my clothes. I started to enjoy getting dressed in the morning. One step in the process was that I emptied my closets of different sized clothes and kept only those that were comfortable and made me feel good about myself. I quit buying clothes a little small, that I could "grow into." Currently I like myself the way I am on most days. This first step was a key to making healthier choices in all other aspects of my life.

Whenever we start something new we take a first step. The first step for better health is to like yourself right now! Stop waiting for that magical day when you will be the right size or shape. Quit putting life on hold until the scale or the numbers let you enjoy life to the fullest.

You can learn to like yourself the way you are. Oh sure, you say: How can I like this lump of clay? Well you can! You can recognize that you are special and unique, a complete and marvelous person just the way you are right now. By changing the tape in your head you turn a negative attitude into a positive one. This change will generate energy, enabling you to choose a healthier lifestyle. Suddenly you'll *want* to make changes to feel better from the inside out.

Heather's words of wisdom and support can apply to you, too, if you choose to let it. But sometimes it's not easy. Penny Muir knows this well, as she shares with you in the next story.

Finding the Courage, *by Penny Muir*

Pearls

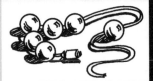

Penny's

It's really tough to accept your body the way it is if you're not ready. I started with my face—in fact, I started with just my eyes. Every morning I looked into my eyes and said the "I like myself, I feel good about myself, I'm going to have a great day" affirmation. Then I moved out to my whole face. I noticed how much prettier, friendlier I was when I smiled. Then I moved out to the rest of me. It was a long, slow process and very difficult to do. When I felt that I was being too critical or unrealistic, I moved back to my face, or my eyes.

Another trick I learned from a teen book on self-esteem. The book suggested taking photos of yourself and cutting off the head so you only see the body. Looking at the headless body gives you the opportunity to be less critical of yourself. I didn't actually try this with a photograph, but I did try it once in the mirror by taping a piece of paper over the spot where my head was and looking at just my body. I really was less critical of my appearance when I couldn't see my head. I don't know why this works, but oddly enough, it does. It is the opposite of the feeling of vulnerability I get when my hairdresser wraps the cape around my shoulders leaving only my head visible.

Something else that I had to do before I could appreciate my body was to make a strong mental note of the good person I am. It was important to identify what I like about the internal me. Realizing that what is on the outside is only the packaging and the good stuff is inside was a real turning point. Now I'm working on revamping the "packaging" so that my inside and outside are a whole.

In her next essay, Christie Keating focuses on a special kind of negative thinking we all are prone to do—the tendency to reduce ourselves to a collection of "problem areas" that need fixing.

My Body or My "Problem Areas"? *by Christie Keating*

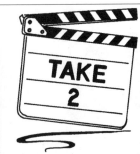

"I just want to flatten my stomach, tighten my buttocks, and firm up my chest!" If we were to enter into an exercise class with this goal, we would be taking a step backwards, into the diet mentality.

Stomach. Buttocks. Chest. These are just body parts.
But is the body merely a holding tank for parts or is it a unit, something to be accepted and appreciated as a whole? By zeroing in on certain "problem areas," we are re-enforcing the message that those parts need "fixing." And if we can "fix" them, then we will feel better about ourselves, and be happier, right?

Wrong.

If we are truly on the journey to better health, we have already learned that it starts first with self-acceptance of who we are *today*. We have given ourselves the permission to experiment to find out what works for us. Physical activity is also part of healthy living. If we are exercising with the hopes of changing parts of our bodies, we are looking for that "quick fix."

The body is a unit, a whole, made up of many muscles, ligaments, tendons, organs, vessels, and veins. Each part has a separate function, but ultimately, they all work together.

Now let's go back to Penny, because she's got something particularly helpful to suggest. Follow her advice and you can get a tidier closet, a better sense of self-esteem, and a chance to do a good deed, all rolled into one!

Cleaning Out the Closet, *by Penny Muir*

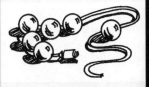

Penny's

Pearls

I've been undergoing some home renovations. I had been clearing out a lot of junk and extras in every room of the house. What a pack rat I am! I gave a lot of dishes and things to charity and it felt so good to do. I had no problem clearing out stuff from every room in the house except for my room, which really started to make me think.

A few years back, as part of the International No-Diet Day celebrations, I had cleaned out my closet and given some of the clothes I never wore anymore to charity. It was a very difficult thing to do. It was actually a lot harder than I had thought it would be. I had decided that I'd get rid of everything and anything that didn't fit anymore and keep only the stuff that fit me at that time. Well, what happened was I gave away only a few things and ended up with my closet sorted in order of size from the current size down to the smallest size I'd ever been. When I look back now, I realize that I had set up some kind of mental measuring table for my lack of success (since I'm nowhere near the smallest, very unrealistic size).

So, during the current renovation process I weeded out old toys from the kids, magazines, dishes, coats, kid's clothes, hubby's clothes, linens, everything. If we didn't use it or need it, off it went to charity. It was such an uplifting thing to do, especially at this time of year. Then I opened my closet . . . and closed it again. I couldn't touch a thing! I think part of me felt that giving away my smaller clothes meant that I was giving up on ever being that size again. Days passed and I kept telling myself it had to be done, once and for all.

So I made a deal with myself. Since the closet was already sorted by size, I'd just get rid of the smallest size, since I knew I'd never be able to hit that size again. Still I couldn't do it.

Then I told myself that since I'm so blessed to be able to be a stay-at-home mom now, and since there are so many single mom's out there struggling to make ends meet, giving away my work clothes would be an extremely charitable thing to do. So I went back to the closet and took out all the work clothes I had that no longer fit me. I had my husband take it that day out of the house and off to the church that collects them for the local women's shelter. It was stressful to do! I can't describe to you how difficult it was to give up that part of myself.

My closet was still jammed full of clothes in various sizes and I really needed to get it cleaned out. It took me four days to muster up the courage to face it again. This time it was just a matter of telling myself that the whole house is fresh and clean and clutter free, except my bedroom and closet and it *had* to get done. So off I went. I sat on the edge of my bed for what seemed like an eternity, just looking at the closet packed with clothes and I felt horrible. I felt that I was facing my biggest failure ever—admitting that I'll never be three sizes, two sizes, not even one size smaller ever again.

I started by taking out everything I currently wear and moving it to another room. All that was left was stuff that I hoped to be able to wear again—"someday"—and

I just folded it up one piece at a time and placed it into bags. I put some stuff aside in a special bag saying I'd keep just *that* bag in storage for "someday."

Hours later, as I stood looking at this perfectly empty closet, I felt so free! I had bags of stuff going off to charity, which is always a good feeling, *and* I was free of the chains from the past. What a revelation! I put back all the clothes I currently wear and sorted them, this time not by size, but by color. I felt so good sitting there looking at my half filled closet, able to see all the clothes I have, and even room to put new stuff in. I felt good about having given so many good and useful clothes to charity, but also I felt released from the pressure of "someday." I truly feel that I'm living in today, for today. Looking at the various sizes of clothing day-in and day-out was exactly the same slap in the face as getting on the scale used to be for me. It wasn't until the stuff was all gone that I realized what a negative impact those clothes hanging there were having on me.

As hard an exercise as it was to do, it was probably the best thing I've done for myself. If you haven't done it, give it a try!

Thin Clothes, Fat Clothes

Like Penny, you, too, can sweep through your closet and remove all the clothes that no longer fit. This closet clean-out will make you feel great. But if you need an incentive to get you started, here's a good one—and one that lets you take an active role in making a difference in your community!

Each year, on May 6, you can join others in celebrating International No-Diet Day by recycling the unwanted clothes in your closet. Stop waiting to get back into clothes that don't fit anymore!

Penny's closet-cleaning builds upon a particular aspect of the diet mindset—the idea of "thin clothes" and "fat clothes." This attitude encourages us to put our lives on hold until we can get back into our "thin" clothes. But by emptying our closets of all those reminders of a former, slimmer size give ourselves the opportunity to begin accepting ourselves as we are right now!

Giving up the old clothes that don't fit you anymore is a symbolic act. It means you've rejected the control that "thin" clothes have had over your life. It means breaking free of the tendency we all have to label ourselves by the size of clothes we wear. So—out with the old and in with the new! Once you've tossed out (or, preferably, recycled) those old outfits, get something new—something that fits you well and makes you feel good! New, good-looking, well-fitting clothes can be a great self esteem booster!

HERSTORY

Getting a Real Life, *by Tanis Rempel*

"What could be more awesome than meeting supermodels Niki Taylor and Tyra Banks, hanging out with TV's hottest soap hunks, and going on a free trip to the most exciting city in the world?" This was the first line of an article about the High School Cover Girl Model Search finalists. The only problem was that, to be a part of this extravaganza, a perfect face and body was an absolute must.

Our society puts a lot of pressure on people to live up to the standards that it has set. Among these standards are beauty, possessions, money, popularity, and fame. Most of us have felt that we were cheated in some department, but there are always those people who seem to have it all. This increases the pressure because, of course, "having it all" is what makes you a respected and admired person.

The age group targeted by the media that is subject to the most peer pressure is the young, and particularly female, population. There are countless magazines that claim to tell you all you need to get your life together and be the perfect person in this society. The problem is that to achieve the necessary standards, young people often go to extremes that are dangerous to the mind and body.

For many young women, the most challenging thing to face is body image. Magazines like *Seventeen*, *Teen*, and *Young and Modern* are loaded with articles on how to enhance your features: How to apply make up, do your hair, and improve your skin. Meanwhile the pages around the articles are loaded with beautiful models that have "perfect" faces. Their faces, however, are not the only perfect things about them. They all are slender, tall, and elegant.

But this is an unrealistic goal for most young people to attain, because no two bodies are the same and you cannot change the basic shape of your body. Presenting so many models who all look the same way creates a tremendous desire to achieve a thin, "perfectly" shaped body. To acquire this "ideal" body shape, many teenage girls starve themselves or practice unhealthy eating habits.

Clothing is another aspect of your image that the media have exploited. The fashion industry really does not help the situation because all of their clothing is designed for those who have slender figures. On the runway, only models with super-slim bodies sport the new clothing, and this just adds to the self-image problem for more normally built girls and women.

Time and again the phrase "be yourself" will appear on the pages of a magazine. However, if you flip a few more pages there is an article about popularity, totally contradicting what they had said about being yourself. The article will be jam-packed with tidbits of information on how to make yourself popular, an absolute must to achieve "coolness." Not so! You can get so caught up in trying to be popular that you lose who you are and become fake. I think that I have accepted the fact that I will never be the popular one in school . . . and I *will not* starve myself—I like food way too much.

People would not be nearly as obsessed with achieving everything society tells us to, if we did not look up to the celebrities in the world and think that they have it all. This is a main goal for young people: to look like the popular actors and actresses, and to someday have everything that they have. Little do we realize that the rich and famous do not have it all, in fact they are a lot further from it than the average person. They may have the possessions, the looks, and the fame, but what about the small things that make life worth living, that give true happiness?

And while teenagers feel a lot of the pressure to conform to society's standards, the older population is not left untouched, either. Carrying the obsession with society's image of beauty with them from their younger years, women still battle to maintain a youthful appearance by fending off wrinkles and using age-defying concoctions. Almost three-fourths of the population of older women do everything possible to retain their youthful appearance. Interestingly, the older models are still taller and thinner than average, but they stress that exercise is the main way to keep them thin and from getting flabby arms. Women get the idea that the actual aging process is unacceptable and undesirable.

I think it is important to be aware of the pressure that society forces on us. If we're aware, then when we're faced with such pressures we will be better able to recognize and deal with them, and avoid harming ourselves or getting caught up in them. By drilling the idea that all of us should look like models into the heads of teenagers, the media are causing girls to harm themselves—sometimes to the point of hospitalization.

It is time that we accept who we are, in image and position in life, and make the best of it by contributing positively to society. We have to drop the obsession to become like the people on TV. They seem to have it all together, but remember, they are actors. Everywhere I look, there is some aspect of society telling me that I should change something in my life, because it does not correspond with the "ideal life." Nothing is left untouched by the desires created by the media or our peers, but I believe that if we focus on the right things, we do not need everything society tells us that we do.

High self-esteem means giving yourself credit for everything that makes you unique, everything that you are. Christie Keating took this truth and came up with a poem:

Me

I see myself as
someone's daughter
someone's sister
someone's mother.
I see glimpses of me.
Just glimpses.
The journey has begun.

Stop Playing the Numbers, *by Heather Wiebe Hildebrand*

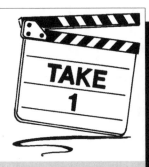

How does shopping around for an outfit at the mall affect you? Here's what happens to me. When I get there I usually feel okay about myself, but nonetheless I enter anxiously, aware of past shopping failures. After a few hours of trying on various articles of clothing, I am so depressed that I go home very grumpy, feeling lousy about myself.

After several months of incorporating the HUGS plan for healthy living, I decided to do a little experiment. Frustrated with attacks on my self-image during each shopping trip, I went into a local mall and made an interesting discovery. I visited approximately 20 different clothing stores, trying something on in each store. Size 15 fit in some stores, but in other stores I couldn't squeeze my big *toe* into a size 15—I needed a size 18 or 20 to feel comfortable. In some shops I could comfortably wear a size 11. This experiment showed that I could comfortably wear a range of 10 different sizes, depending on the store in which I found the outfit. No wonder my perception of my size and shape were affected when I went shopping!

I am not the only person affected by these size discrepancies. I have a friend who is 5 feet 2 inches tall and very petite. She went into one store and discovered that the only tights she could fit into comfortably were a size Large. She left that store thinking that she needed to lose weight—she saw the "L" on the tights and decided that meant that she was huge! She *believed* the label. But did fitting into a size Large mean that her size and shape had changed? Of course not. Still, she allowed the size label on the article of clothing to dictate how she felt about herself.

The labeling inconsistency sets another trap that I have fallen into when shopping for clothes. I would end up buying only my regular size, regardless of how the clothing fit. Then I'd hope that this new outfit would motivate me to change my size and shape. I put my life on hold, until I could fit into the right size. This tactic never worked, but it *did* keep me from feeling good about myself.

People have allowed the fashion industry to dictate how they feel about themselves. They become very discouraged when they go into a store and discover that they suddenly do not fit into their normal size. Often they will be depressed for days and their self-image suffers. But individual sizes and shapes do not change in a day. So, what is going on here?

Stores—and clothing manufacturers—have different sizing strategies, depending on their target market. For example, stores that cater to the teenage market tend to have clothes with a tighter fit, while expensive, exclusive shops have clothes that fit larger shapes—and they label these items to flatter their targeted customers.

The time has come for us to challenge the fashion industry's sizing practices, but more importantly the time has come to quit letting the fashion industry's sizes dictate how we feel about ourselves. The numbers on clothes, just like the numbers on the scale, are poor indicators of how we actually look. We need to quit using the external numbers around us to determine how we feel about ourselves. Once we realize how little those numbers actually mean perhaps we'll be able to take the next step and disregard them.

I challenge each of you to go shopping and try my little experiment. You can see for yourself how the numbers and sizes vary from store to store. They are a very unreliable indicator for success or failure in our process to better health. We need to find more reliable indicators of better health. Internal indicators that are more reliable include increased energy levels, healthier attitudes toward food, enjoyment of activity, improved self-image, and internal feelings of health and wellness.

Climate and customs in North America regulate our need to wear clothing. Thus, we have to access the fashion industry, regardless of its discrepancies. I encourage you to find clothing that is comfortable and makes you feel good about yourself. Find outfits that suit you and your style. You want to enjoy today, and to do this you need to feel good about yourself. As Naomi Wolfe observes in *The Beauty Myth*, how we look is easily influenced by how we feel about ourselves. If we feel good about ourselves we tend to look great. Appearances come from the inside out. It is time we stop paying attention to external numbers. You and I know they don't really mean anything after all.

Heather knows that you don't have to take what society and, particularly, the beauty industry dishes out. You can find your own standards and live according to them. Here's an allegory by Heidi Mead that makes this point very well!

HERSTORY

Riding High and Free, *by Heidi Mead*

Imagine yourself doing something you've always dreamed of doing—like riding the biggest rollercoaster, taking a dream holiday, relaxing with friends and family, or getting in touch with nature. These things all can make you the person you want to be. They can also just allow you to become the best you can be.

So—instead of imagining—DO IT! Just get started, and it will come true. Now it's time to get organized and let the dreams start taking over. That's what I did. I decided to move toward my goal: started packing, got some friends together, planned the menus, did the shopping, packed up the scads of equipment—then headed out for a weekend of paradise!

Here is the scene: Perfect blue sky, the weather is warm, the water is warm, the wind is calm, the moon is out, and everyone is enjoying the sights: eagles, turning leaves, brilliant reflections on the calm water, stars glimmering in the sky, the moons of Jupiter visible through the spotting scope, and the sound of owls, herons, and other night creatures surrounding us. We're all taking this chance to get away in September to soak up the best that Lake of the Woods has to offer. We've planned and fantasize about what our sailing adventure will bring us tomorrow! This could be paradise, we think.

Then, the next day dawns: Cloudy, windy, and cooler. We need to pull out the jackets, sweatshirts, and rain gear. Oh well—this can happen to the best laid plans. And just imagine: now we've got great winds to carry us anywhere we want to go! So all right! Let's get packing! If we wait for perfection we might miss the most memorable times we could ever have. And besides, that's what sailing—and life—are all about: opening up and grabbing on to whatever you are presented with. Going with the flow! Is this paradise?

We pack up the boat and get on board. Everyone has their places, with Captain Russ at the tiller; Second Mate Mitchell learning about the boat and what he can do; Third Mate Linda taking her spot in the middle so she can stay dry and help with the sheets; and First Mate Heidi on the bow, ready to hoist the sails or take them down as necessary. We head off on a reach, southwesterly, and plan on sailing toward the open water to challenge the wind and the water with our trusty boat, which seems more like a whale ready to play and get some exercise.

First things first: we all need to practice tacking and getting the hang of the come-about, which takes only a couple of seaworthy attempts before everyone is proficient at it. We even enjoyed heeling over (riding at an angle) and looking at the keel as it nearly rises to the surface while the boat is taken to great speeds by the wind. Onward, we all decide—this is going to be great! (Getting close to paradise? Perhaps.)

As the boat continues out of the bay, we start to realize the wind is much stronger than we had thought, so we decide it is time to reef the main sail. We find a place to do it that is not too much into the wind, but the task requires teamwork and cooperation. And of course, being friends, and experienced, this is accomplished without too much squawking and bustling about on the boat.

Once again we head off toward the open water and the high rolling waves. We soon discover the waves require us not only to hang on and ride hard, but also to don our rain gear—warmer clothing to really meet the true excitement of the wind and the waves. We gather speed (and some water) as we head to what we hope will be a sandy beach for lunch. But alas, after rounding an island, the wind strikes us with such force and enthusiasm that we decide to head for one of the biggest and most southern islands we can get to. We're thinking that this will allow us an opportunity to dry off and calm down.

"Ha-ha!" cries the wind. "I have you now!" We reach the island only to find that the wind has us surrounded and there was almost no where we can get off. But with the steady and experienced hand of our mighty Captain Russ, we manage a docking against a sheer cliff at which the most hearty sailor would have marveled.

On land at last, we replenish ourselves with delights that people can only dream about, all provided by master planner Linda. After regaining our energy, our sense of adventure takes hold of us once again, and we decide to head north—back to our home base, and what we hoped would be more polite waves.

Little did we realize the wind was going to be our tour guide again: we were greeted by waves that nearly dwarfed the boat! We had thought it impossible to encounter a more invigorating ride on the wild side than we had experienced on the trip out, but Mother Nature had a surprise for us! Forget Disney World and other water parks—we had our own non-stop, gale-force rollercoaster ride, complete with howling winds, crashing waves over the bow, and drenching water breakers.

We sneered! We laughed! We called to the wind! We even dared it to get *more* intense! We felt as one, riding the crests and breaking over the rollers together! Nothing could daunt us as we sailed toward home, confident of our abilities and the steadfastness of our boat. Nothing could beat us! Our Captain was flawless and we trusted his skills completely.

We roared along at speeds not often seen with sailboats at Lake of the Woods, almost as though we possessed a new-found energy that allowed us to break free from the common world. Everything was tingling and real—everything was so tangible! It felt so good to just live and to feel what it was like to be one with the elements. It was almost like Mother Nature herself was calling to us to come and play. (Does this seem like paradise? I think we are getting closer.)

We survived everything Mother Nature gave us and felt satisfied with the sail. We all felt we had the time of our lives, riding high and free, with only the thought of being here and now on our minds. The whole experience wasn't what we had planned or how we dreamed we would spend our time sailing. And we could have decided rollercoaster waves were too much for us, but we had decided to tackle the odds and rise to the challenge. Because of our wild and free attitude we enjoyed a once in a lifetime experience. It wasn't based on who we were or what we wanted. It wasn't based on being in control or planning for the right event—it was just being free enough to let ourselves enjoy and experience the best that was offered to us. (That sounds like a kind of paradise.)

We learned, we laughed, we roared, we shared, and most of all we *were*. Life and sailing are like that—what is real is the best. Learn how to savor and immerse yourself in what is real—and *enjoy*. Everything has value and should be savored. Allow yourself to experience the whole and you, too, will be wild and free! (Paradise!)

Taking It Deeper

- **On: The Scale Moves Around But I Stay the Same**

  1. Have you lost a substantial amount of weight in the past? Discuss how you felt after people stopped noticing?

  2. Did the weight loss change who you were, how you felt, how you dealt with crisis?

  3. If you've ridden the diet rollercoaster, how many ups and downs did you experience? Discuss your past weight-loss experiences, sharing both your positive and negative feelings.

- **On: Who's in Charge?**

  1. Take a closer look at the questions on the quiz. Although you're supposed to answer the questions honestly according to your present reality, would your answers have been different at other times in your life? Discuss why your answers may have changed.

  2. If you have difficulty becoming the decision-maker in some areas, ask around and see what others do. Evaluate their responses and discuss how they may (or may not) work for you.

  3. In some instances, we may willingly choose to have someone else make the decision for us. And that's OK too. Do you have such instances in your life? Discuss why it is sometimes appropriate to delegate decision making in those instances.

- **On: Ten Steps to Loving Your Body Just As It Is**

  1. Review the ten steps and discuss how you are applying them to your life.

  2. Go down the list and identify the ones that you have already put in place and are working for you. Discuss the ways that taking these steps have made a difference in your self-esteem.

- **On: Change That Tape in Your Head (or Discoveries from a Soup Bowl)**

  1. Heather notes that "creating a positive self image is probably the biggest challenge most people face . . . . I still have days when I struggle with my self-image and outward appearance." Discuss Heather's comments and how they may apply to you.

  2. Heather notes that slipping into negative thinking every once in awhile is normal, but that it is important to notice this and take steps to turn it around. What strategies does Heather use to accomplish this? What additional strategies can you suggest?

- **On: My Body or My "Problem Areas"?**

  1. Try Penny's body-assessment technique: Start with your favorite body parts, look at them, enjoying the way you look, and then move onto other parts so that you can learn to admire them as well.

  2. Penny notes that when she's at the hairdresser and they drape the cape around her shoulders so that only her head is exposed, she feels "really odd, sort of vulnerable and exposed." Discuss why she might feel this way. If you share her reaction, examine you own feelings and the reasons for them.

- **On: Cleaning Out the Closet**

  1. Why was the closet-cleaning exercise so important to Penny? Share her experience by tackling your own closet and getting rid of clothes that no longer fit, then discuss how it made you feel. If you find it difficult to toss out those old clothes, discuss the reasons why.

  2. Cleaning out your closet may make you feel so good that you want to take a more active role in making a difference in your community. If you're in a support group, take on the Recycle Your Closet Campaign for International No-Diet Day (INDD) on May 6. Go to www.hugs.com and put your own local campaign together. We want to hear about your plans to make this vision a reality. Take a stand and make a difference!

- **On: Getting a Real Life**

   Tanis writes, "You can be so caught up in trying to be popular that you lose who you are, and become fake." Discuss how the pressures and obsessions you faced in your own adolescence may still carry over into your life today. Consider how they may have contributed to diet thinking in your life.

- **On: Stop Playing the Numbers**

   1. How do you feel when you buy something that fits and looks good on you? What action will you take to do this more frequently?

   2. Have you noticed that a range of clothing sizes fit you? Try Heather's experiment in your own local shopping mall.

   3. We aren't completely under the control of the fashion industry's sizing policies. Here's an exercise that lets you fight back locally: When shopping in a store that divides up women's clothing according to "extra sized" and other euphemisms, make a point of using the customer comments card (available at the service desk) to bring your displeasure to the attention of management.

- **On: Riding High and Free**

   1. Have you got a personal vision of paradise? Using Heidi's story as an inspiration, try writing down (or talking about) your own vision, and what you might do to make it become a reality.

   2. Heidi's sailboat was a vehicle to experiencing freedom. What would your own "sailboat" be?

Getting Back into Exercise 8

Exercise According to the Experts
Diet Thinking about Exercise
Are *You* Diet-Thinking about Exercise?
Exercise Gives Back, in Droves
Pace Yourself!
The Tortoise Wins the Race
Exercise, Dieting, and Metabolism
Exercise, Like Oxygen, Gives Energy

I s that gym membership going unused? Is your tennis racket shoved in the back of the closet with other dusty exercise equipment? In this increasingly sedentary culture, exercise is something we all know we should do, but often don't get around to. Or we yo-yo exercise—get all gung-ho for a few weeks or months, then drop out.

As important—and arguably *more* important—as what you eat is how much you exercise. Piles of research papers point to the same thing: fitness is the key to longevity, good health, and well-being. I can't stress enough the value of exercise; it's so important that I've devoted two chapters to it!

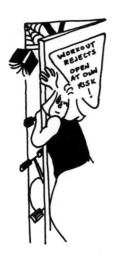

Exercise According to the Experts

For those of you who struggle with exercise, there's good news from the research front: you don't have to do intense exercise to stay healthy. A year-long study published in a 1999 issue of the *Journal of the American Medical Association* found that people who accumulated about 30 minutes of activity daily by raking leaves, taking a brisk walk around the block, or taking the stairs instead of the elevator, improved their blood pressure and other measures of heart fitness just as well as those on a structured exercise program. And they were even *better* at maintaining a healthy weight.

And other research shows that breaking activity into chunks—such as two 15-minute walks—is just as beneficial as going for 30 minutes straight. So, for those of you who feel like skipping this chapter because you can't bear to read about hour-long aerobics classes, stay with me. Your 15-minute walk to the lunch spot near your office is already doing you a world of good.

And there's even better research news for those of you struggling with your weight: you don't have to lose weight to reap benefits from exercise. In an ongoing Duke University Medical Center study, mildly obese men and women maintained their body weight over a three month period, while exercising four times a week on a treadmill, stationary bike, or stair exerciser. Preliminary results published in 2000 found that although body weight didn't change, people lost fat and gained muscle, which heightened their metabolic rate. Their "bad" LDL cholesterol dropped, while levels of "good" HDL cholesterol rose.

We have come a long way from the days when being fit meant being thin to the realization that as long as you are fit you are healthy, no matter what your body size. If you look in today's bookstores, you'll find a wide array of self-acceptance and nondiet books—the tide is turning. People are starting to speak up, and starting to make friends with their mirror. In fact, the television series *20/20* ran a story on this very subject, showing people of all proportions being physically active and enjoying it. The focus of this story was feeling better, and health was defined by energy level, blood profiles (that is, blood sugar and blood cholesterol), and blood pressure. Yeah!

This is the kind of information that we need to hear more about in the mainstream media. It makes it easier for us to stand our ground against the diet mentality. Can you just imagine when you get the next crack about your weight saying, "Didn't you see the "Fit and Fat" story on *20/20*?" You have the edge. What a nice change!

"Good" cholesterol (HDL, or "high density lipid" cholesterol) actually helps your body rid itself of build-ups in cholesterol levels. "Bad" (LDL, or "low density lipid") cholesterol, on the other hand, just sticks around to increase your risk of heart disease!

And how about the new slogan: "Health at any size." It describes a movement that meets people where they are in their health journey. It's a celebration of seeking health enrichment without focusing on weight or size. Does this bold claim seem to leave you out of the picture because you're presently inactive? Well, don't worry. With self-improvement—not perfection—as your goal, you are ready to join the movement, believe it or not!

So, how do you get back into physical activity? What's absolutely essential is that you find some form of exercise you like, even if it doesn't burn a zillion calories. If you've been a dieter, why not take all that determination and energy you've been putting into dieting and—one step at a time—divert it to the movement of your body? Take it slowly, gradually, and without imposing an overwhelming time commitment on yourself: That's the key that unlocks the door to lasting change.

In order to feel confident about who we are, we do need to take some responsibility in being active and healthy. We can't just become couch potatoes and say "accept me as I am." Read on for some tips that will make it easier to get started, whether it's for the first time or the hundredth time. And some pointers on how to make this new activity a lifelong habit.

Diet Thinking about Exercise

"I ate a doughnut. Now I need to wear off the calories by going for a walk for half an hour."

Or

"I walked to the doughnut shop. The doughnut is the reward for the exercise I did. Calories in/calories out . . . that is what I was always told."

If these thoughts sound familiar, you may have transferred diet thinking over to your approach to physical activity. But your goal is to banish the diet mentality from your approach to exercise. Here's a quiz that rates how much of your attitude toward exercise is influenced by a diet mentality. Each column in the quiz describes a different exercise habit or attitude toward physical activity. If you relate best to the attitude that appears on the left, put a check mark in the leftmost column. If you relate to the attitude on the right, put your checkmark there instead.

Are *You* Diet Thinking About Exercise?

	Are You "Diet Thinking" About Exercise?		
	I exercise because I know I should—after all, I know what's good for me.	I like to exercise. I enjoy myself and have fun.	
	I'm not walking unless I've got a destination in mind.	I like walking for the invigorating fresh air and pleasant scenery. It's a relaxing time.	
	When I eat a forbidden food, I try to burn off the calories with exercise—I guess it's punishment for doing the wrong thing.	I take time for myself by living actively.	
	After I've exercised I tend to reward myself with food.	I've found that just the simple act of participation in physical activity is enjoyable and rewarding to me.	

	It's normal to feel stiff and sore after exercise. If it doesn't hurt, it can't be doing any good. Don't they say no pain, no gain?	When I exercise for a period of time, I include warm-ups and cool-downs.	
	If I'm not wiped at the end of the exercise workout, then it isn't worthwhile.	I have discovered that exercising to the point of energy and not exhaustion has regulated my appetite.	
	I'm exercising to lose weight, but I always get a strong enthusiastic start and then peter out.	I'm comfortable about the amount of exercise I do. I feel more fit, energetic and self-motivated.	
	Exercise is just one more task on my "to do" list	I'm taking slow steps forward with putting physical activity into my daily living.	
	I've got to fit in my exercise at the end of the day.	I anticipate my physical activity. I view daily decisions such as moving wood, carrying in parcels, and using the stairs as valid activity.	
	I really take exercising seriously. I'm into speed and power walking as often as possible.	I like to be consistent and regular with my exercise.	
	When I'm huffing and puffing during exercise, I know it's working.	It's important to me to be able to carry on a conversation during physical activity.	
	I play to win; that's what sport is all about.	I enjoy my sporting activity, it's a fun and social time for me.	
	Exercise is really a waste of time; I like to be productive.	I have found that exercising actually gives me time. With my elevated fitness level I'm more productive and efficient about doing more in less time.	

How to score:

Add up your checkmarks in the right hand column—that is your score in the nondiet-thinking category.

Over 11: Congratulations! You're definitely hooked on activity!

Over 7: You're well on your way to appreciating enjoyable activity for fun.

7 or less: Re-read the nondiet column. You'll find plenty of cues about how you can move into nondiet thinking about exercise.

If you've got lots of checkmarks in the left (diet thinking) column, you will want to examine how your mental attitude affects your approach to physical activity and think about how you might make some changes.

Like the Diet Mentality Quiz, you might want to retake this test periodically to get a sense of your progress in changing your attitudes toward exercise over time. The more you get away from the diet mentality, the more your score should improve.

Exercise Gives Back, in Droves

The World Health Organization describes health as "a state of well-being, of feeling good about oneself, of optimum functioning, of the absence of disease, and of the control and reduction of both internal and external risk factors for both disease and negative health conditions." Without fitness as part of your regular life, this definition is unlikely to describe you.

On the other hand, a fit body gives you a state of well-being. It makes you feel good about yourself, your physical accomplishments, and the way your body moves. For this you can thank, in part, the mood-elevating endorphins that kick in during and after exercise. Mental health is a by-product of being physically active, whether it's a relaxing stroll or a power walk, yoga or a step class. To some degree, in other words, exercise is as much about making time for clearing your head with physical "me" time as it is about a workout.

And, in so many ways, exercise makes your body function better: you're less likely to be constipated and your body becomes more responsive to insulin, keeping blood sugar at a more even keel. Exercise protects your heart in so many ways: by lowering blood pressure, raising levels of "good" HDL cholesterol and strengthening the heart so it pumps more blood to the rest of the body with each beat.

By learning what it takes to be active, by observing and by adopting as your role models others who enjoy being active, you can begin to make a very important contribution to keeping yourself healthy and independent. How can you afford *not* to do what it takes to become active? Just keep this simple equation in mind:

Regular Activity = Energy

So let's get going!

Your first step to becoming more physically active is to pick something you enjoy. As Penny Muir puts it, "For me, exercise is the last thing I'm putting in my new lifestyle. I'm starting to swim laps because I enjoy it, it's not strenuous, and it is a solitary activity which gives me the time I need for me. I just turn off for a bit and lose myself in the activity. The thought of doing it for any other reason would send me into resistance or rebel mode."

Think there's no exercise that you could enjoy? Think again. Here's a list of activities that might jog your memory. Make a check mark next to the types of activities you'd like to do and those that seem possible for you right now. Indulge your fantasies— what would *you* like to try? Think about the aspects of the activity that you find appealing. For example, Jane explained it this way. She recently heard someone describe the exhilarating feeling of parasailing (flying behind a high-speed boat!). Now, that was not for her, but it got her thinking about the joy of free movement, the wind against her body. She thought, "Maybe it's time to add variety to my beloved treadmill walking."

- ☐ Aerobics, regular
- ☐ Aerobics, low-impact
- ☐ Ballet
- ☐ Baseball
- ☐ Basketball
- ☐ Curling
- ☐ Cycling
- ☐ Dancing
- ☐ Football
- ☐ Golf

☐ Gymnastics

☐ Hiking

☐ Hockey

☐ Jazz

☐ Jogging

☐ Lawn bowling

☐ Martial arts

☐ Racquetball

☐ Roller-blading

☐ Rowing

☐ Sail boarding

☐ Skating

☐ Skiing, cross-country

☐ Skiing, downhill

☐ Skipping

☐ Soccer

☐ Squash

☐ Swimming

☐ Swimming, long distance

☐ Tai chi

☐ Tennis

☐ Volleyball

☐ Walking

☐ Water-skiing

☐ Weight Training

☐ Yoga

I'm confident that you can find at least one thing on this list that you'd enjoy doing. And don't be intimidated by an idea just because you haven't tried it before. For example, weight training isn't hard to do: You're basically standing or sitting the whole time, and you pick your own weights, so you can start out with very light ones.

Pace Yourself!

So how do you find your stride in fitness? Well, just like everything else we talked about so far, it is a process that takes experimentation, time, and a recognition of the limitations set by your present fitness level and body shape.

Let's say you've decided that some indoor activity is best for you. Your choices might include dancing, swimming in an indoor pool, going to a gym (if you prefer some type of socialization), or investing in some type of fitness equipment that you can use at home. You make your choice—or choices—according to what you realistically feel you can do on a regular basis.

Some choices require more self-discipline than others. Working out at home, for example—whether it's stepping on that treadmill or popping in an exercise video—requires lots of self-motivation. But after awhile you may find that you look forward to the wonderful feeling you attain during and after the exercise. That feeling is the exhilaration of a heart pumping faster, the satisfaction of hanging in there even though it's not as fun as being out cross-country skiing or tennis, and the energy level attained from regular physical activity.

So how can you get to this point? I can only tell you how it worked for me. Here's my story:

Normally, I love to ski. But one winter was really harsh, and my opportunities to go skiing were limited. I began to feel very lethargic—my energy level was very low and I had little motivation to do anything about it.

As spring set in and I began to be more active again, I paid attention to how nice this felt. I started thinking ahead to *next* winter. I didn't relish going to the gym several times a week as I do enough traveling already and am usually just happy to be home. I also did not care to work out along with others unless some outdoor activity was involved. So I began looking around and trying out different equipment, and decided that the treadmill was for me, especially because walking is one of my favorite activities.

So I got myself a treadmill. When winter came along, I just got on it and used it, right? Not quite. Any new piece of exercise equipment takes time to get used to, especially for someone like me, who really prefers to be outdoors. I had to find a way to learn to like the treadmill. Here's how I did it (and these tips will work for an exercise bike or any other piece of aerobic equipment as well):

- Take a gradual approach. Take the first five minutes slowly, then build up a momentum for a period of time that keeps you energized (not exhausted). Then slow down for the last five minutes for your cool down.

- Try interval training. You plug in your rest speed and work speed, and the treadmill alternates the speeds so that you maintain your heart rate without working so hard that you're killing yourself. Just as you are feeling a little tired for example, the machine switches to your rest speed so that you can keep on going without wanting to give up. In my experience, this also keeps my treadmill time more interesting.

- Make it a priority. Make exercise a part of your regular routine, not just an add-on at the end of your day. Otherwise it's very easy to leave it out.

- Get into focus. Tune in to your body and note the difference that regular activity makes. Even though exercising may not be your favorite way of getting active, recognize that it's improving your feelings of well-being.

As you really get into becoming more active, you may want to try including some additional types of activity for variety. Living in Canada, where the winters bring plenty of snow, I alternate between cross-country skiing and using the treadmill. I'm planning to get myself a pair of snowshoes next—I tried snowshoeing a couple of years ago and have been thinking about it ever since. It took two whole years to move that thinking process to action—I finally made the decision to actually do it by reasoning that, where we live (out in the country), snowshoes will actually come in handy, making wintertime outdoor chores so much easier.

And, of course, when the weather turns warmer, there are other activities that might tempt you. Long bike rides in spring and fall can make a wonderful break in your days. Hiking in the woods or simply walking into town on a pleasant day can lighten you mood as well as help you get fit. And if you have access to a lake or stream, why not consider swimming or rowing in the summertime?

One other way to increase your activity level is to spend time with friends who enjoy being active too. The buddy system can add to the pleasure of the experience, because it adds a social dimension: While you're walking or skiing you're also talking or just enjoying some quiet time together. And there's always the pleasure of indulging in some pre- or post-activity fun, like getting together afterwards to enjoy a hot drink.

The Tortoise Wins the Race, *by Penny Muir*

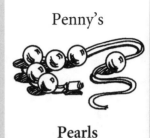

Penny's

Pearls

Getting excited about exercising is great, but don't get so carried away that you overdo it. You'll regret it later. Here are two walking scenarios that will show you what I mean.

Scenario 1: You start out with a fast-paced power walk, pushing yourself as hard as you can, huffing and puffing through the whole walk so that your arms and legs feel like jelly when you're done. The next morning everything hurts—but you're determined, so you go out again to walk. But either you stop halfway through because it just hurts too much, or your mind starts playing those awful berating messages about being too big, too out of shape, and so on. So you quit and go home. Or you stick it out and finish the walk, but by the time the next day rolls around you're so stiff and sore that you just can't take another walk no matter how much you want to. Instead, you take the day off, and maybe even the next day. Now you have to start all over again, and you've spent the last few days listening to those horrible messages about yourself, so you're fighting an uphill battle now.

Scenario 2: You decide to take a leisurely half-hour stroll around your neighborhood. You set out, and you admire the scenery. You're just wandering along, your mind wandering as well—you don't even know *how* much time has passed and poof, you're home again. You're not huffing and puffing, you're not sweating—but you *do* feel invigorated and relaxed. You get up the next morning and you feel the same as you do every other day: NO PAIN. So off you go again on day two. Same thing—you stroll along, enjoying the sights, smiling at some passersby. Again, before you know it, you're home. Again, you feel invigorated. The messages in your brain are positive because you're proud of yourself for being out two days in a row and you have no pain.

On day three it rains and you decide to skip your walk. You notice that, unlike your experience of the past two days, you haven't had a chance to clear your head, so you realize that even after just two days, the walks have been doing some good. So you decide that, rain or shine, on day four you're going again. Before you know it, you've become so accustomed to that half hour stroll that you feel miserable if you don't get it in. Perhaps a friend joins you and, because the pace is manageable, you can actually enjoy each other's company. Maybe the kids come along. Before long, you realize that you have more stamina. You may even have picked up your pace. After a very short time you're noticing a change in your attitude and your ability. Your attitude has changed because you made a fitness plan and you stuck to it. You're getting fitness benefits because you're *still* doing it.

The point is, that while the pace of the walk in scenario 2 is much, much slower than the power walk of scenario 1, you'll be doing the slower pace more often. It's like the tortoise and the hare fable—slow and steady wins the race. You don't burn out, you're enjoying your time, you keep going. If you don't enjoy it, you stop; what benefit have you gained? And that's when the messages start playing in your head "I'm lazy, I never stick to anything, I'm hopeless." Also, if you go into it full force, with a lot of initial passion for it, somewhere in your brain you expect to see "results." When those results don't materialize right away, you're liable to become disappointed and quit.

Exercise, Dieting, and Metabolism

I have been asked this question a few times: Since exercise counteracts decreases in metabolism caused by cutting calories, why not combine diet and exercise? The answer is simple: when you diet, you focus on weight loss. Chances are, however, that effort involved in weight loss will lose its charm, and your new diet and exercise lifestyle will be temporary. For it to become a lasting change, the process toward fitness must become the internal motivator—it's far more reliable than using the external motivator of a weight-loss goal. In addition, even though physical activity increases your metabolism and offsets some of the effects of dieting, it doesn't offset those effects completely. That's because, while exercise increases your metabolic rate by around 10 percent, dieting decreases that same rate by 15 to 30 percent, so there is still a net metabolic deficit of between 5 and 20 percent.

HERSTORY

Exercise, Like Oxygen, Gives Energy, *by Shelley McDonald*

Fitness is for everyone. I am adamant about the right approach to incorporating activity into your life. Now, do you think I'm Miss Fit, hanging around the gym munching energy bars. Not! But I am fit, strong, and healthy. I have that instant energy I need to reach my 5-year-old before his sticky fingers touch the new couch—the kind of energy we all need to get through a busy day.

I exercise at home whenever I can, preferably when my two-year-old is still sleeping—it's impossible to do a sit-up with a 25-pound toddler sitting on you.

And I incorporate a fun activity into my day whenever possible. We don't need gym memberships, we need to take the stairs. We need to stand, not sit. We need to walk, not ride. Take some deep breaths, sending that oxygen to every cell, every tissue. That's what oxygen is, a fuel source—as important as food. You've heard of anaerobic. That's when you're out of breath, red in the face, pushing the oxygen out, not taking it in.

Our sedentary lifestyles only require shallow breathing. I'm not giving up my garage door opener but the truth is unless we're looking to be active we don't have to be. We don't need to breathe deeply to do our work, but our bodies still need that oxygen. Try taking a few deep breaths, really filling your belly, sending the oxygen racing to the ends of your toes and fingers. I'll guarantee you that you will feel a little more energetic, a little more alert, and a little more focused. Try it! You might like it!

To exercise is to oxygenate your body. So let's exercise and let in that energy-giving oxygen. But remember, you have to build up to a fitness level. It's potentially harmful and no fun to go for a walk with a friend or into an aerobic class and try to keep up with someone who has a higher fitness level than you. Build yours! But don't do it because it burns calories. Do it because it feels good. Find something you really like to do, and then *do* it. The payoff is energy and endurance and strength.

When exercising, keep in mind form, control, resistance, and always, always modification. You can do movement all day and never change your body. If you move properly once, you *will* change your body.

Believe me, when I first recognized the difference between "dancing" aerobics and truly muscle-building, fat-burning aerobics, it was just like a light bulb coming on. Whether you're doing aerobics or going for a walk, you need to use the natural resistance in your body. For example, you can move your arm up and down in one of two ways. You can just swing it up and down, or, using your natural resistance, you can *press* your arm up and down. You can let gravity do it, or you can make your body do it. And when you make your body do it you are building muscle strength.

Now try stepping from side to side. Same thing: just stepping, or *really* stepping. Pressing your heel down and pulling your other leg over to meet it. If you do it you will feel the difference. You can imagine you're pushing through mud or water or against a beach ball if that helps. And now you're moving properly using resistance, control, form, and most importantly modifying the exercise if it gets to be too much. You want to get that energy source (oxygen) into your body, you don't want to be gasping it out. If you are moving properly within your fitness level you will feel good. You will have energy and you will continue to build to a higher fitness level. Best of all, you will continue the activity because it makes you feel good and gives you energy.

We are whole beings. Wellness is not just physical but mental and spiritual as well. Olympic gold medallists don't just train physically. The sports psychology they use is just as available to each of us. If you *see* yourself as fit and healthy, eventually you *will* be. Most importantly, know that you don't have to go it alone.

Taking It Deeper

- **On: Exercise According to the Experts**

    1. How does being active fit into the goal of health at any size? Without being active, can you really say you are healthy?

    2. Describe the images that the phrase "fit and fat" conjures up in your mind.

    3. Research shows fitness is the key to health and longevity. If you are active, discuss the process that worked for you in getting to this point.

    4. If you are presently inactive, think about activities you enjoy and the steps you need to take to become active. Make a list of the steps and check them off as you put them into action.

- **On: Diet Thinking about Exercise**

    Using the quiz as a starting point, discuss how diet thinking has affected your ideas about physical exercise. Focus on those areas where you have successfully overcome the influence of the diet mentality, as well as on those areas where you could stand some improvement.

- **On: Exercise Gives Back, in Droves**

    1. What does fitness mean to you? Examine your definition, and be on the look out for diet thinking.

2. List the mental benefits of physical activity.

3. List the physical benefits of physical activity.

- **On: Pace Yourselves!**

  1. Describe a process that would help you to make some form of physical activity work for you in your own climate conditions.

  2. Discuss one or more types of physical activities that you might be interested in taking up and the strategies you might use to take yourself from thinking about it to actually making it a part of your everyday life.

- **On: The Tortoise Wins the Race**

  1. Contrast Penny's scenario 1 with scenario 2. Discuss how they differ, and examine why one approach is more likely to result in long-lasting change.

- **On: Exercise, Like Oxygen, Gives Energy**

  1. As Shelley says, we do live in an overly complicated society! She suggests that we remember to breathe fully. How is this suggestion helpful? Give her tip a try, then examine how and why it works.

  2. Shelley identifies three tools for defeating the diet mentality: food, fitness, and fun. She also identifies three payoffs: energy, endurance, and strength. Using this essay and the one entitled "Passion Ignited" in Chapter Three, examine how Shelley uses all three tools to beat her own diet thinking.

  3. Discuss Shelley's discoveries about the effective use of oxygen and the role of natural resistance techniques in physical activity. How can you apply these techniques to your exercise routine?

126

Making Exercise a Lifelong Affair

9

Sticking With It
Everyday Exercise
Bob's Breakthrough
The "Shoulds" of Exercise
Putting the "E" (for Enjoyment) into Exercise
Exercise Is *Not* a Dirty Word

K, now you've found an exercise you like. How are you going to make it stick this time? I've got three tricks that will help:

1. Keep trying new forms of physical activity so you don't get bored.

2. Along with—or instead of—programmed exercise, incorporate more movement into your everyday chores and activities.

3. Work on shifting your attitude so that exercise becomes something you cherish and enjoy, and not a dreaded task.

The goal you want to achieve here is to eventually make fitness so much a part of your life that it's like brushing your teeth regularly—if you miss out on it one day, it kind of feels yucky. Your body needs to be lubricated with movement just as your teeth like to have that sparkling clean feeling. Pay attention and be sure that you tune into how your body feels and relish the moment. The tips and personal accounts in this chapter will help inspire you to make exercise a lifelong companion.

Sticking With It

There are certain things you can do that will help you stick with physical activity for life. One is to avoid going into activity full force and then stopping cold turkey. If you a start an activity gradually, you are more likely to make it a long-term habit. An off-and-on approach to activity, on the other hand, simulates off-and-on dieting attempts. In addition, when you go into exercising whole hog from the start, there is bound to be some muscle pain. After the first few times you'll find that you have to stop until your muscles stop hurting. Then you'll have to start all over again, so you'll start to wonder "why bother?"

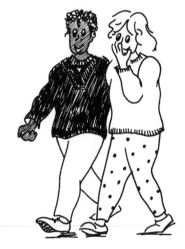

A better way is to think of what you like to do, start visualizing yourself doing these activities, and then begin saying positive affirmations to move that thought into action. Make everyday activities part of your fitness plan: gardening, a trip to the market, a short walk, vacuuming. They all count.

It's also wise to protect your fitness time. Make it a regular part of your daily schedule. If you don't—if you treat fitness activities as something you just tack on to your day whenever you've got some free time—you're likely to start skipping it, until you've dropped it altogether.

There are lots of other ways to help keep yourself on the fitness track. For example, you can start making friends with people who enjoy being active—you'll support each other in the process of enjoying the way your body moves. And you can try a variety of activities, noting which ones make you feel good. This will help you to want to repeat the process, to want to do more. Any diversion of this sort from regular activity can totally rejuvenate and inspire you.

Also, realize that *everything* counts. Be sure to grab onto any opportunity that you have to get moving and keep moving. And balance your lazy days with action—if you anticipate a sitting day tomorrow, be sure to get moving today. Similarly, balance spectator activities (watching a baseball game, for example) with activities that make you part of the action: golf, walking, and hiking.

But avoid thinking of physical activity as a chore. Instead, use your activity as a social time where you can walk and talk with a close friend and ponder the day's activities or reflect on your upcoming projects. The idea is to pace yourself: Build in a balance of moving activities like walking, tennis, aerobics, cycling that keep your blood circulating and make you feel good and healthy. On the other hand, be careful not to get too active, which can leave you exhausted rather than energized. Split your activity up into small intervals. Remember that two 15-minute walks are just as beneficial as a 30-minute walk.

If exercise increases your appetite, you may be working at too high a level. High intensity exercise depletes your carbohydrate stores (glycogen), and that post-workout hunger is a signal to refuel for energy. This type of exercise leaves you exhausted. If exercise dampens your appetite, then you are working at the level right for you. This level of activity leaves you feeling energized and raring to go. Make sure you drink fluids to rehydrate yourself. If you are working at a level right for you and are still hungry, you may need to rehydrate yourself first with fluids. If you don't, your body will signal "hunger" in an attempt to get those fluids from food.

Most of all, know and accept your limitations. Don't expect to be able do your activity every day when you haven't been active for years. Make a plan to do your activity only a few times a week at first, and build in a plan to increase it by one time every few weeks. Here's how Penny got her exercise plan off the ground—see if you can use some of her tips to develop a plan that will work for *you*!

Everyday Exercise, by Penny Muir

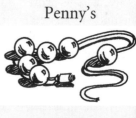

Penny's

Pearls

When you think about adding a little movement to your day, do you think only of "exercise"? Does this idea conjure up images of sweat and pain and little enjoyment? It did for me. Then I realized that it didn't have to be some regimented plan of sit-ups, jumping jacks, and stationary biking in order to be beneficial.

I started out by making a list of the activities I liked to do, inside or out, rain or shine. What I came up with was a variety of activities I could do and enjoy. This list included swimming in my local pool, walking and biking along the miles of trails near my home, and dancing in my living room to the music I love to listen to.

I loved the solitude of the walks and bike rides. They allowed me to enjoy my surroundings while actually hearing myself think. The swimming allowed me to clear my head and think of nothing at all. Then I started taking my young daughter along on some of my outings. This is when I realized how much muscle training I was doing and what an aggressive, relentless personal trainer I have in my daughter.

When she joined me on my walks when she was young enough and co-operative enough to stay in her stroller, I would pick up the pace to her chants of "faster Mommy, faster" until I found myself actually jogging for parts of the journey. When I took her along on my bike rides, the ride was never long enough for her. Now that she is 3-years-old, she's too big and too bold to stay in a stroller or bike seat, and I find that our walks are as fast as her little legs will take us. Once we are at the park I discover myself lifting her 3 times, 9 times, 100 times up to the top of the slide, up to the monkey bars and down again. Just imagine the upper body strength!

My personal trainer/daughter's favorite activity is what she calls "silly dancing." The sillier the better. Just when I think I have had all I can take, there is my daughter begging "one more time Mommy. Pleeeeeeassssssse?"

And I have found that bedtime to her is actually stair-master time. One trip upstairs for a drink of water, and down again. Another trip upstairs to take her to the potty, and down again. A trip upstairs to make the scary things go away, and down again. Another trip upstairs for more kisses, cuddles, and tucking in, and on and on and on until one of us finally collapses. I'm sure that every parent has experienced the kind of personal training my 3-year-old is dishing out.

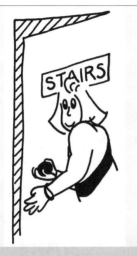

What I had thought would be the hardest part of my new lifestyle turned out to be the most enjoyable. Think about it. How can *you* add a little more movement to your day? Make a list of the activities you enjoy. Take a look at your daily routine. What changes could you make? Here is a list to help you get started. Make your own additions and try to make one change in your routine every week. You may be amazed by the way you feel.

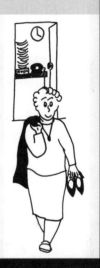

- Park a little farther from the entrance to the office or the mall or the grocery store.

- Get off the bus a block or two before your regular stop.

- Walk the children to or from school instead of driving them.

- Take the stairs instead of the elevator.

- Add a little more vitality to your housework by turning up the music *you* like and moving to it. Who is going to see you?

- Take a walk at lunch instead of staying at your desk and working through.

Bob's Breakthrough

A couple came over for a visit on a wonderful snowy day. It was perfect weather for cross-country skiing. We only had two pairs of skis—my own and my husband's, and I asked Bob if he wanted to try cross-country skiing with me. His initial comment was "I don't like cross-country skiing—it's not as exhilarating as downhill."

But Bob went ahead and gave cross-country a try—and found a new kind of exhilaration. He could now spend some time in conversation with his friend while skiing, creating some special sharing moments—something he could never do on a downhill ski run. This isn't to say that downhill skiing is not enjoyable and exhilarating—it is and it does have many benefits. But each type of activity has its own perks and benefits, and Bob was discovering the joys of cross-country that he never recognized before. He was actually taking time to enjoy the scenery. He was even working some newly discovered muscle groups. All-round, he experienced a consistent and peaceful, playful time that was not only fun but also was a great activity that would help improve his fitness level.

Try putting aside your own preconceived notions and give new types of activity a chance, like my friend Bob did. Really exploring a new activity with someone who thoroughly enjoys it can make all the difference. Only then can you begin to grab onto the excitement of the particular activity. As you begin to enjoy and explore and experiment with different types of activity, you'll acquire the desire and confidence to want to try more.

The "Shoulds" of Exercise, *by Heather Wiebe Hildebrand*

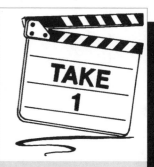

Vegetables are a colorful, multi-textured, versatile food group. They are high in fiber and vitamins and low in fat, and many are an excellent form of complex carbohydrates. Many people view vegetables as a necessary food that you "should" eat. Healthy eating means including more vegetables in your diet. This idea is often approached with low enthusiasm. But when people start to view vegetables as an exciting part of a meal, to be enjoyed and prepared in many different ways, they begin to crave them and choose them willingly.

Many of us view activity or exercise in the same light as vegetables. Something we "should" do to become healthier. Active living has been a big struggle for me. Even after taking a ten-week HUGS course, I still had difficulty making activity a fun part of every day living. How could I adopt activity into my life as a natural and fun part of my day? How do I make activity a desire rather than a "should" or an "ought"?

I have found that exercise has fallen into my diet mentality almost more completely than my eating habits. I have used the all-or-nothing attitude toward it: If I can't walk for forty minutes, I may as well not even go out. If I don't have time to reach my target heart rate, what's the point of working out?

After some reflection I have made some discoveries. There seems to be two problems linked with activity and permanently integrating it into my lifestyle. One is "I just don't have the time" and the other is "I really don't enjoy activity."

Here's how I have worked through the time dilemma. In the past I have seen activity as something that requires time slots in my day. In my mind, activity was something that I should do to become firmer and more slender, and to achieve a healthier body. I also felt that activity needed to be scheduled and routine in order to be effective. Often I didn't have the time during my day to book an hour of aerobics, or take a trip to the gym for racquet ball. When I didn't have the time I would just do nothing and this made me feel I led a sedentary life, an exercise failure!

In the process of reviewing my activity and lifestyle, I have looked back at my grandmothers. They had less time than I do, with thirteen children and farming tasks. They never booked a special hour to be active. I think that is because their whole life was active, without even trying. They lived to healthy old ages by being active and enjoying life.

Some may argue this is because they didn't live in a fast-paced, automated world. Well, that is true but I think we can learn from them. They always took active routes to complete their activities of daily living. We need to learn to make these choices as well—with ideas like parking a little further away from our destinations so that we can enjoy the walk, using the stairs instead of the elevator, playing street hockey with the kids, bringing the walking shoes to appointments or noon hours to fit in some quality shopping or walking.

Time doesn't always allow us to fit in long hours of activity, but it often allows us moments where we can enjoy the most active route to a task. My husband's grandmother is an inspiration to me. She is one of the most vital women I know. She wakes up every morning and massages her arthritic limbs and stretches so that she can move during the day. She makes sure that walking and movement are part of her daily routine. She walks with friends, works for hours in her garden tending her lovely begonias, and enjoys many hours quilting in her basement, walking up and down the stairs to keep herself limber. She is one of the happiest, healthiest women I know. She loves life, and she is 84. I hope to be more like her! For her, being active is a gift, something to be treasured and enjoyed.

My second problem with exercise is: "I just don't enjoy activity." But I reviewed this statement and began to evaluate why I felt this way. Could it be my all-or-nothing attitude, where the focus is on numbers rather than the benefits and joys of activity?

Being obsessed with numbers takes all of the fun out of an activity for me. If I do activity because I "should," I easily become tired and overwhelmed, and soon I feel like I never want to do that activity again. When I changed how and why I was active, however, my views shifted. I started to enjoy the process (being active) and quit focusing on the end (target heart rates, covering a certain distance, and so on).

Like every new habit, I first learned about it, practiced it, and finally affirmed myself in the process. I stopped focusing on how long I exercised or how far I ran; I consciously turned my mind to other things. Every time I thought about the calories I was burning or how much further I should be going I tuned into how my body was feeling right at that moment, and I talked about it out loud. If I was with someone, I told them how the activity was making my body and mind feel. I intentionally focused on what was around me and commented about that.

It takes continuous practice to change a habit like the focus of exercise. Over time, I have found that I enjoy activity more and more. I've come to miss activity when I don't take the time to include it every day. I have become more and more creative at fitting activity into my lifestyle. I am learning to choose the most active route, and you know what, it's *fun*.

I have realized that my attitude toward activity is what determines if it will be a positive or negative process in my life. As long as I treat it as something I "should" be doing to become healthier, I will not be able to incorporate it as a fun part of my every day. I need to change my focus. You may need to do this as well.

But it takes practice to change your focus. We all have days that we slip back into the numbers game. Don't let that get you down, just acknowledge the slip and keep going. Affirm yourself on how far you have come and tune into your response to the activity. Choose the most active route and have fun.

Putting the "E" (For Enjoyment) Into Exercise

The key to becoming a "repeat exercise customer" is to make it fun. Use these ideas to make active living work for you:

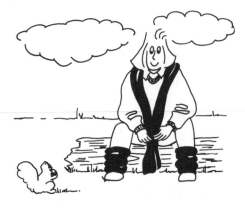

- Rather than focusing on the numbers of how far, how high, how long, focus on your surroundings, and how your body feels before, during, and after activity.

- When you go for a walk, start making a conscious effort to notice your surroundings.
  - What pictures are you seeing?
  - Who are you with?
  - What are the smells, sounds and textures around you?
- How does it feel to have your heart pumping and your face warm with the vitality that fresh air gives? Do you feel energized at the end of the activity?
- Focus on the enjoyable parts of activity; you'll be more likely to come back for more next time around.

HERSTORY

Exercise Is *Not* a Dirty Word, *by Christie Keating*

We all know that exercise promotes healthier bodies and minds. So it only makes sense that we should increase our present level of exercise. Nike ads say "Just Do It." I say, "sounds great, but what is it we're supposed to be doing, and how do we do it?"

Let's first take a look at the word "exercise." Exercise is a word used mainly to describe a particular function. For example, doing abdominal exercises works the abdominal muscles of the body. To say that you're going to an exercise class implies that you will be working different parts of the body's muscles, including the heart, using the standard format of warm-up, cardiovascular exercises, cool-down, muscle exercises, and stretching.

As a fitness instructor, this is the format that I use. However, at the risk of losing some of my participants, I would like to challenge this notion. Or at the very least, stir up some discussion. Is exercise the only way to a healthier body? What about other forms of physical activity? To me, the term "physical activity" implies being physical with an activity. Makes sense, don't you think?

But I think the real difference between exercise and physical activity is our own perception. One is not necessarily superior, just different. There are people who enjoy the format of a class, the feeling of exercising a particular muscle. There are also individuals who are more apt to enjoy walking, cycling, or swimming. The real issue is to find an activity that you enjoy.

Exercise and physical activity are on the same health continuum, they just occupy different spots. Respect and understanding for each would help eliminate the "one is better that the other" attitude. After all, your healthier body is still the goal, and if you're having fun, well, that's even better. Just remember—*any* physical activity or exercise is beneficial to your health.

Taking It Deeper

- **On: Sticking With It**

    1. Work through each of the "keeping exercise interesting" points, examining how they may work for you.

    2. Discuss the efforts you make to protect your fitness time and keep it from becoming "add-on" at the end of the day that gets squeezed out.

    3. Select an activity that you might enjoy and try visualization (imagining yourself actually doing the activity and enjoying it) as a way to overcome any fear or resistance to making it happen.

    4. Learn to listen to your body—pay attention to the signals it's sending you as you engage in physical activity. Remember, your goal is to exercise for energy, not for exhaustion. When your exercise level is appropriate, your body will reward you with a sense of renewed energy.

    5. Think about where you are now with regard to physical activity and what your goal is 3 to 5 years down the road. Lock on to that goal and outline the steps you'll need to take to get there, one step at a time. Be sure to pace yourself so that you don't fall back into that all-or-nothing thinking where you end up going into the activity too full force only to peter out and say that it's not for you. Share this process with others, if possible, and team up with a buddy who shares your goals.

- **On: Everyday Exercise**

    1. Discuss the everyday life activities that Penny does. Note the process of building more activity into her lifestyle.

2. Examine Penny's practical list of suggestions that are designed to give you a little push on your own activity levels. Select two or three and examine them for their potential usefulness in your own life.

3. Discuss the following statement: "What I thought was the hardest part of my lifestyle turned out to be the most enjoyable." Apply it to a time or event that happened in your own life.

4. If you aren't regularly active yet, examine what you need to do to move from talk to action?

- **On: Bob's Breakthrough**

    1. Discuss how Bob changed his perspective on an activity just by trying it and observing his friend's interest in the activity.

    2. Give examples of people you know who are enjoying various activities that you have not tried yet. Find out what makes them enjoy it. Consider asking one (or more) of them to introduce you to the activity as well.

- **On: The "Shoulds" of Exercise**

    1. Discuss Heather's two obstacles to being more active, and examine her solutions to them. Identify obstacles that you face to increasing your activity and the steps you might take to overcome your own.

    2. Heather closes her essay with the comments "I need to change my focus. You may need to do this as well. It takes practice to change your focus. We all have days that we slip back into the numbers game. Don't let that get you down, just acknowledge the slip and keep going. Affirm yourself on how far you have come and tune into your response to the activity. Choose the most active route and have fun." Discuss how these comments may be helpful in fighting "all-or-nothing" thinking.

    3. Examine your relationships to identify whether they are nurturing—helping you achieve positive growth—or negative. Discuss how the attitudes of the people around you may have an effect on your own sense of satisfaction in life.

- **On: Exercise Is *Not* a Dirty Word**

    1. Discuss how you perceive the difference between exercise and physical activity? Is the difference truly all about perception?

    2. Make a list of your present physical activities. Discuss how you might expand this list with new activities that you've always wanted to try but never gotten around to doing.

Tuning into Hunger and Thirst

10

Reclaiming *True* Hunger
Eating to Hunger: How to Eat
Take the Guilt Out of Eating
Snacks: Guiltless Pleasures
Hunger-Staving Snacks
Quenching Your Thirst
    Water, water, everywhere
    What's enough
Tuning into Thirst
    Water before meals doesn't work
    Debunking diet drinks
Carbohydrates Need Fluids

Y ou can't have a healthy relationship with food until you learn to respond appropriately to your hunger and thirst signals. And establishing a healthy relationship with food is at the core of the philosophy of this book, at the core of getting and staying off the diet rollercoaster. Years of dieting (even if you've stopped dieting for a while) may have impaired your responses to hunger and thirst. You eat when you're not hungry, or you let yourself get too hungry because you're *afraid* to eat. You eat when you really need to drink, or you can't even tell when you're hungry or thirsty anymore. Don't worry, it's all damage that can be repaired. This chapter offers some tips on how to do that.

Reclaiming *True* Hunger

What does it mean to feel hungry? What does it mean to feel full? Those were easy questions to answer when you were a child, and experienced those sensations naturally. But soon the assaults on hunger set in. For instance, family conditioning can make you feel bad about having "too big" of an appetite, or you're served meals that are out of synch with your hunger. Then there's dieting, in which you try to *conquer* hunger, followed by bingeing, in which you surpass hunger. All of these derail your hunger signals. But when your hunger and satiety (feeling full) signals get back on track, you're on the road to improving your relationship with food.

These phrases probably sound familiar to you:

- "Better watch what you eat unless you want to become like me."
- "Clean your plate or you won't get dessert."
- "Finish your meal—people are starving in . . . ."
- "Don't spoil your dinner by eating now."

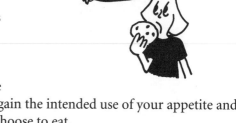

Those are the kind of reactions most of us received when we expressed our appetite. But appetite is normal—celebrate this simple body cue with pleasurable nourishment instead of suppression. Here are some suggestions that can help you regain the intended use of your appetite and consequently start to enjoy the food you choose to eat.

- Identify hungry and full feelings.
- Start a pattern of fueling your body regularly every four to six hours.
- Eating breakfast will make you hungry at lunchtime—a natural and desirable effect.

Respond to your hunger feelings by eating. It sounds too simple, I know! But if you ignore your body's signal of appetite, you're apt to have cravings—and you'll possibly binge later on. That's because, if you come to the table feeling completely famished, you'll gobble down too much food without even tasting it. So, plug in a light snack when you are beginning to feel hungry—even if it *is* just before a meal time.

> How much to eat? Eat for energy, not exhaustion!

And here's another "too simple" tip that really works: When you are full, stop eating. The skill of re-determining when you are full will emerge over time. You can help it along by adopting slower eating patterns, taking time to chew each mouthful. You'll discover that sometimes you won't be able to eat everything on your plate!

Eating To Hunger: How To Eat?

You may do best on three square meals every day; others need a snack or two in addition to breakfast, lunch, and dinner. And grazers are most content with about six mini-meals daily. All of these patterns are perfectly healthy as long as the foods are well chosen. As far as what to put on your plate, well, despite the extremes prescribed in fad diets—no carbs, only cabbage soup, only fruits—research supports one basic type of diet. This way of eating has room for variation.

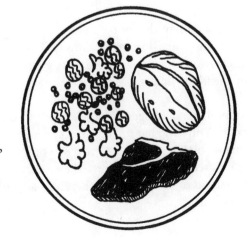

As you can see in the picture the basic eating plan consists mainly of carbohydrates like whole grains, potatoes, rice, pasta, fruits, and vegetables. These foods take up two-thirds to three-fourths of your plate. The rest is protein such as fish, poultry, meat, cheese, soy, or other vegetarian equivalents. As you begin to tune into taste and texture of naturally low-fat foods such as fruits, vegetables, and whole grains, you won't need as much fat. *Fat becomes a way to accent, rather than mask, your meals.*

Carbohydrates fuel your body with immediate energy, and protein helps regulate appetite, helping hold you over until the next meal. To find the exact proportions that are right for you, keep experimenting to find the perfect balance. Don't be fooled into taking "dieter fare" like a soup and salad combo for lunch—it has too little substance to sustain you and simply sets you up for a 3 o'clock binge. Add a sandwich to that soup or salad for a lunch that will bring you closer to the evening meal without feeling famished.

The important thing is to abandon diet thinking and its distorted eating and behavior habits. Feed your own appetite and relish each mouthful!

> Here's a quick rule of thumb for creating a meal that's nutritionally balanced and helps stave off hunger. Visually divide your meal plate into quarters or thirds. One-quarter to one-third is protein. The other three-quarters or two-thirds are carbohydrate-rich foods, either starches or fruits and vegetables. You can play with these carb quarters (or thirds) as fits your needs. Divide them equally between starches (such as bread, rice and potatoes) and fruits and less starchy vegetables (such as greens, cauliflower, and the like). This balance of food types will provide holding power, a feeling of fullness and satisfaction, and energy for hours of activity. This carbohydrate and protein balance is critical to providing a sustained sense of fullness that prevents cravings.

Take the Guilt Out of Eating

Taste and savor the food you have selected. Don't spoil your enjoyment of the food by telling yourself that you shouldn't be eating it. This is diet thinking and not a celebration of food. Your aim is to become physically and psychologically satisfied by the food you eat.

Make dietary changes slowly. Let's say you usually order a large plate of fries with gravy. You love that mushy, greasy feel, but you may be just as satisfied with a smaller plate, without the gravy, if you experience the texture of the crispy, gravy-free fries and tune into their taste. You haven't made a radical change and gotten rid of the fries altogether, instead, you're tailoring your taste away from some of the fat.

Focus on the texture and taste to see if you can appreciate the difference. Penny Muir says "I have found out that by savoring a mouthful of Maple Leaf Fudge, I actually don't like it as much as I thought I did! By focusing on the taste, texture, and enjoyment of the favorite food, it may not be all we thought it was."

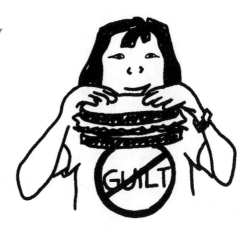

Remember that it takes time to move away from familiar food combinations; if you give them up as a matter of discipline instead of preference you're apt to develop a craving and feel deprived. In Chapter 12, "Tailoring Your Tastes," you'll learn how to make those gradual changes. For now, we'll concentrate on the first step: getting back in touch with your body's own hunger signals.

Snacks: Guiltless Pleasures

Snacks—the little extras in life. The bites that tide us over to the next meal or help us make it through the night. Snacks have a bad reputation, but remember, they can fall anywhere on the nutrition continuum. Snacks can be sweet or salty, or simply leftovers from yesterday's meal. Some snacks are quickly grabbed fast foods, others are intricately prepared, elaborate morsels.

Some of you may be afraid to keep snack foods in the house, afraid you'll wind up overeating. But barring them from your house may make you binge on them later on. Think about it: what happens when there is nothing you like in the house? Do you wind up standing in front of the buffet table at the next social event eating those very same "forbidden" foods? Or even eating them under the covers when you're alone?

Eating healthier does *not* mean never having chips or a chocolate bar. It means enjoying them when you really want them, not living off them as a central part of your daily food intake. Remember, by forbidding foods, you can become obsessed with them. If you stop eating the foods you love, in time you'll pig out on them. It's no fun to be always thinking about food, so snack when you really want to, and enjoy it. You will actually be satisfied with less—remember, you don't have to eat it all if you don't want to.

Hunger-Staving Snacks

When balancing your daily food consumption, snacks provide exciting little time outs, supplying your body with the nutrients it needs to physically survive and become healthy. But how do you know when your body needs a snack? Here are some questions to ask yourself:

1. "When did I last eat?" Was it more than three to four hours ago? After several hours your body needs to be refueled.

2. "Am I really thirsty instead of hungry?" Your body sometimes sends hunger messages when actually it's liquid that it wants. Before eating, check out the effect of having something to drink—a spritzer made of fruit juice and sparkling water or lemon water. Does this remove the hunger? If it does, you were probably just thirsty. But this doesn't mean that you should use the dieting trick of drinking great volumes of liquids to mask your hunger. Fluids are meant to rehydrate the body. Says Penny Muir, "In the beginning, I found that it was easier to tune into hunger than to thirst. Now I can tell the difference between the two, but when I'm rushed for time, hunger still comes through louder than thirst."

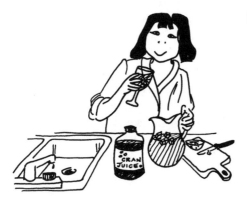

3. "Am I feeling symptoms of lowered blood sugar?" Low blood sugar can give you headaches, shakiness, weakness, difficulty in concentration, and other symptoms. If you're experiencing these symptoms, chances are your body is crying out for some energy foods. Don't ignore your body! Learn to listen to it and answer its needs.

4. "Am I bored, tired, or upset?" Sometimes you'll feel this way because you're hungry, and a snack will do the trick. But even when these feelings have nothing to do with hunger, they can still drive us to food. Then we eat, and we're still bored, tired, or upset. So we eat again; clearly setting a destructive pattern. By addressing our feelings by trying some form of stress relief other than eating, however, the hunger feelings might dissipate. The importance of giving yourself

"time outs"—little perks—cannot be stressed enough. We all need time to rejuvenate mind, body, and soul. We need fun spontaneous moments in life.

When should you take a non-food time out and when should you snack? The snack should be in response to *real* hunger. Otherwise, take a walk, read a book, call a friend, or treat yourself to some other form of time out. You know you need it when life becomes so hectic that you can no longer cope with the little things. When you find yourself unhappy with the tasks that you need to do every day, when you are bored, when you feel bitter and angry all of the time, or when you no longer feel like you are worth anything and you quit looking after your body and mind. If you experience any of the above, then time outs are essential. Do something for yourself, something that adds spice to your life or something fun or silly or something that helps you to grow.

Balance Means Taking Snack Times, *by Heather Wiebe Hildebrand*

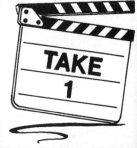

I remember drilling the words "You have to avoid the snacking times if you hope to lose weight" into my diet memory. Snacks received careful planning to stay within daily limits. Snacks were the ultimate in diet "sin."

I used to equate snacks with extra calories. Today, however, snacks are a very important part of my daily life. They provide "time outs" where I can rejuvenate my body and my mind.

After monitoring of my body's needs, I discovered that there were days when I was hungry between meals. My body required extra food or fluids in order to function optimally. Researchers have suggested that many small snack meals are actually healthier for the body than three larger meals. The more constant availability of food gives a steadier amount of energy for the body to draw upon and reduces the feast-and-famine response in our bodies. Learning how to snack has helped to reduce the number of times I would lose control in the area of food consumption.

When working the day shift as a public health nurse, I would be starving by the time I got home at 5:30, but wouldn't eat then, so as to save room for supper. The result was a grumpy woman who prepared much more food than two people could eat. I also nibbled while preparing supper, and then wolfed down a huge meal at the table. I regularly felt stuffed.

Since then I've developed balancing skills which allow me to listen and respond to my body's needs. I felt better when my routine changed. When I got home, I would sit down for about 5–10 minutes and enjoy a light snack—a piece of fruit, or fruit-topped yogurt, or a few crackers—and unwind a little. After unwinding I'd start cooking dinner. I felt more relaxed, enjoyed the preparation period, and no longer ate while preparing the food. At the dinner table I was able to gauge the balance of carbohydrates and protein I need to sustain a healthy body.

A pre-dinner time out provides the body sustenance as well as a mental and emotional break. Balancing activity, work, fun, relaxation, and spiritual time is essential in coping with life and its stressors. Disregard for balance in any area triggers old eating and coping patterns that are very destructive.

Changing my daily patterns to eat a snack that rejuvenates my physical body has been fairly easy. However, incorporating time to rejuvenate my mind and soul has been more difficult. I spend hours doing things for others but I have trouble justifying time out for myself. I feel selfish when I spend time just for me, especially if it is for fun or relaxation. But this really isn't selfish at all. By giving and giving without rejuvenating, I rob myself of time needed to heal, grow, and rebuild. I slowly become an ineffective helper.

A common problem in the "helping" professions is to spend years caring and giving only to end up bitter and resentful. Professionals who become snappy and short tempered are very ineffective in the caring department. We can all run out of the energy to give, and when that happens our bodies and souls resort to self-preservation. Effective care-givers take time out for themselves. Time spent rejuvenating physically, emotionally, and spiritually can be the "snack" you need to restore a healthy, well-balanced perspective in life.

Quenching Your Thirst

Are you thirsty? If so, you may already be a little dehydrated. Probably even more common than losing touch with hunger is losing touch with thirst. The human thirst mechanism isn't the greatest, that's why by the time many people feel thirsty, they're already dehydrated.

Drinking enough water—whether your thirst tells you to or not—will help you stay off the diet rollercoaster. For one thing, drinking liquids helps to regulate your food intake. People often mistake thirst for hunger and eat when what they're really trying to do is quench thirst. When your body is dehydrated it may send out hunger signals because there is water in food. And it's not always fruits and other watery foods people turn to, sometimes they will even eat more of foods that do not contain much water—foods such as meat. Obviously, it's best to satisfy thirst with fluids. A hydrated body is a happier, healthier body, and that's always a plus when you're trying not to diet.

You may be surprised to know that 55 to 60 percent of your body weight is water. This is the natural balance. Water that is lost through urine or perspiration has to be replaced—that's called the rehydration process. Other factors that affect the water level in your body include the menstrual cycle, your diet, your exercise level, certain medications, and even the weather—you lose water through perspiration on hot days. Salt and carbohydrates cause the body to retain water, which is why eating lots of salty or sweet foods can make you feel bloated.

Water, water, everywhere

You know, you just can't live without water! And for good reason, because water:

- Increases energy and endurance
- Helps to digest meals
- Helps to get rid of waste products via urine
- Regulates body temperature
- Gives us a feeling of well-being
- Acts as a lubricant for the limbs and joints so the body can stretch, twist, and flex itself
- Helps to maintain proper muscle tone by giving muscles their natural ability to contract and by preventing dehydration
- Helps relieve constipation. If the body has too little water, it gets what is needed from internal sources. The colon is a main source of extra water. If water is pulled from the colon (part of the intestine), then you end up with a hard stool—constipation. When a person drinks enough water, normal bowel function returns.
- Flushes your system and hydrates your skin—both important for healthy looking complexions.
- Reduces risk of kidney stones
- Linked to a decreased risk of colon cancer, probably because it dilutes cancer-causing substances in the colon and flushes them out quickly.

What's enough?

Think that daily three cups of coffee, the diet drink you have at lunch, and that glass of milk with supper are doing the trick? Sorry, you're still short on liquids. Women need eight or more glasses of liquid a day to maintain normal body functions; men need about twelve glasses. Liquids should quench your thirst and replenish the water stores in your body.

But certain liquids are actually de-hydrating. Coffee, tea, and alcohol are examples of dehydrating beverages. (Ever notice how they cause you to run to the bathroom more frequently?) Even decaffeinated coffee and tea contain other stimulants that are dehydrating. And soft drinks don't truly quench your thirst because they remove more fluid than they provide. Here's why: while beverages like soft drinks add fluid to the body, they also add salt and sugar, substances that must be diluted as they enter the bloodstream. When the concentration of sugar and salt increases, your body first tries to dilute them by pulling fluid from the cells into the bloodstream. But that fluid is soon lost forever in the urine. At this point, you feel thirsty again—the increased concentration of substances and diminishing fluid content triggers your thirst mechanism. Plus, pop and drink mixes like lemonade, iced tea, or juice made according to package directions often leave a sweet taste in your mouth, leaving you thirsty and still drinking.

Diet drinks may have these sugar substances removed, but all caffeinated beverages —including caffeinated soft drinks—remove water from the body by affecting the hormones that regulate your fluid balance, thus causing your system to produce more urine. And besides, from a health point of view, diet drinks may not be your best choice of liquid.

Water is your best choice for quenching your thirst and for rehydrating. It is ready to use and doesn't contain sugar or chemicals that the body has to process while extracting the fluid. But many people don't like the taste of plain water or tap water and won't choose it when they want a drink. If you're in that camp, here are some things you can do to learn how to retrain your taste buds and give plain old H_2O a chance:

- Add some sparkle. Mixing sparkling water into your favorite drink or punch will heighten the flavor and add fizz. While some sparkling and mineral waters contain some sodium (salt), many don't. Check labels: Many brands of plain and flavored seltzer and sparkling water are salt-free.
- Add plain or sparkling water to dilute fruit juice.

- Add more water to powdered or crystal beverage mixes than what's recommended on the label.
- Add sparkling water to a glass of your favorite soda pop. Start by adding one-fourth cup of water to each cup of soda.
- Add extra plain milk to chocolate milk to make it a little weaker. Also, try easing down from whole or 2 percent milk to milk that's lower in fat— low-fat milk contains more water. (See Chapter 12, "Tailoring Your Tastes," for the best way to ease down on the fat content in your milk.)

As you make these adjustments to your beverages ask yourself these questions. By trying to answer these questions you'll begin to discover beverages that satisfy your thirst and are better hydrators.

- How does the beverage feel in your mouth?
- Does it quench your thirst?
- Does it add to your body's water stores?
- Does it taste good?
- Does temperature make a difference?

Tuning Into Thirst

You can train yourself to become a better "thirst sensor." For one thing, you can start paying closer attention to what your body is telling you with its hunger signals. When you think that you feel hungry, drink some fluids first—before you turn to food. If, after having that drink, your feelings of hunger subside, then that hunger signal was merely your body's way of prompting you to take in more fluids.

On the other hand, if you're feeling hungry and you haven't eaten in three or four hours, and your mouth doesn't feel dry, then there is a good chance that you really *are* hungry.

While you're retraining yourself to recognize your body's request for more liquids, try being creative in coming up with satisfying thirst quenchers. For example, you can add water to drinks or juice to make it into a taller drink—one that makes you feel like water is literally being pulled into your body. Don't believe me? Try reaching for plain or slightly flavored water one day when you are really thirsty— you can practically *feel* your body's cells soak up that fluid!

Water before meals doesn't work!

You often hear people say that if they drink water before meals they won't eat as much. But this only works for the short term. Here's why: Water fills you up quickly, making you feel bloated and giving you the sense that you have less room for food. So you eat less; maybe even not enough to really satisfy your hunger. But a little while later you're hungry again—because you didn't eat enough in the first place.

You can temporarily fool your body into thinking that you are full by drinking water before your meals, but watch out! Your hunger eventually catches up with you. Remember your body needs food for energy.

Debunking diet drinks

Diet thinking has never been more obvious than in the marketing of diet drinks. Every restaurant, diner, and fast-food outlet carries them, and there's a 50–50 split between diet and nondiet drinks on the supermarket shelves. Even people who say they are *not* on a diet often pick diet drinks. I'm sure you've noticed people who'll select a huge piece of cake or order a large plate of fries with gravy—and then wash it down with a diet drink because "the drink has no calories!"

We tend to believe that drinks that are traditionally served ultra cold—like milk, milkshakes, lemonade, or beer—will quench our thirst better than warm or hot ones, but that's often an illusion. They may taste and feel satisfying, but do they really rehydrate us? You'd be surprised!

Take milk, for example. An icy-cold glass of milk sure seems thirst-quenching, but it doesn't do a very good job of adding to your body's water stores. That's because the high calcium and protein content in milk requires your kidneys to use some of your body's stores of water to process it.

Milkshakes are another example of a drink that's traditionally served cold but that isn't permanently thirst quenching. A high-sugar drink like a milkshake actually keeps you thirsty and the milk in it, once again, requires water from your cells to process the calcium and protein. Don't believe me? Next time you order one, notice how it feels in your mouth.

Carbohydrates Need Fluids

Your body always needs water, but water is particularly important when you're eating carbohydrates such as whole-grain breads, pasta, and rice. Carbohydrates are stored as glycogen in the liver and muscles—and they are stored *with water*. Foods like whole-grain bread also contain fiber, which pulls water from your cells like a sponge. If you don't drink enough fluids, the fiber in these foods won't function properly in their task of moving the food through your intestine. In other words, you may end up constipated.

Keep this fact in mind if you're trying to increase your fiber intake. Add only a bit of fiber at a time, and make sure to increase your water consumption at the same time. Otherwise you'll find that too abrupt an increase in fiber will make you feel bloated and may cause gas.

What to look for	Why this happens
Dry mouth, thirst	The body's initial response to dehydration when you lose up to 1 percent of your body's normal water weight.
Dark urine, small urine output	Water is the main ingredient in urine, which transports wastes from your body. When you're dehydrated these wastes get concentrated because your body tries to hang on to all available water. This causes your urine to darken.
Headache	This is a sign that your brain is short of oxygen. Oxygen is carried by blood, which is mostly water.
Swollen hands, feet, and legs	Water is normally stored in your cells, but when your body is trying to protect its water level it needs extra storage space—like a pantry. The body picks spaces outside the cells to store this saved water, which causes these areas to swell.

What to look for	Why this happens
Rapid heartbeat; weak, fast pulse	Since blood is mostly water, dehydration means you have a diminished supply of blood. When this happens your heart races to pump this diminished supply of blood to your muscles and organs.
Dizziness, confusion, difficulty in concentrating	When your blood supply is diminished, there's less for your body to pump to your brain. This reduces the amount of oxygen and nutrients available, causing dizziness and impairing your ability to think or concentrate.

Taking It Deeper

- **On: Reclaiming True Hunger**

  1. Consider the following phrases: "Better watch what you eat unless you want to become like me;" "Clean your plate or you won't get dessert;" "Finish your meal—people are starving in . . . ;" and "Don't spoil your dinner by eating now." Discuss these phrases and suggest ways in which you can respond to them.

  2. Over the next few days, make a point of trying to ensure that you eat breakfast. Discuss how including this meal affects your hunger level throughout the day—particularly how it affects the frequency with which you experience hunger feelings.

  3. Make a list of some of the signals you recognize when your body's trying to tell you it's hungry. Discuss what happens if you wait too long before eating: do you tend to eat more? Do you eat more quickly? Do you eat until you feel over-full?

- **On: Eating to Hunger: How to Eat?**

  1. Now that you're trying to keep to a regular schedule of mealtimes and working to develop a good balance between carbs and proteins,

keep a mini-log of your hunger sensations over the course of the day. When you note a true hunger signal, try a light snack and then make note of how it affects your ability to come to the next scheduled meal feeling pleasantly hungry, not starved.

2. Experiment with different carb-to-protein combinations, and note the difference in your body's hunger signals four hours after eating.

- **On: Snacks: Guiltless Pleasures**

1. When you register a hunger signal, allow yourself a guilt-free snack. Then discuss the effect that this has on your ability to approach mealtimes with a good, but not excessive appetite.

2. Examine the effect that guilt-free snacking has on your mood, self-esteem, and sense of well-being.

3. Next time you treat yourself to a favorite food, take time to consume it slowly and savor every mouthful. Examine your body's response: do you find that you need more or less of the food to feel satisfied? Does your actual experience of the food live up to your anticipation of the treat?

- **On: Hunger-Staving Snacks**

1. Discuss the ways that snacking can serve as a "time-out" to re-energize your body. What other things can you do to make yourself feel pampered?

2. Evaluate your current approach to snacking. Do snacks "spoil" your appetite or help control it?

- **On: Quenching Your Thirst**

1. Genuine thirst is one of the most overlooked signals in the body. Monitor your own thirst signals and discuss how you can determine whether they indicate thirst or hunger.

- **On: Water: Why You Can't Live Without It**

1. What are the reasons you can't live without water?

2. Discuss the causes of dehydration and how the rehydration process works.

- **On: What's Enough**

  1. Which fluids are dehydrating, and why?

  2. The next time you find yourself experiencing a true thirst signal, pay close attention to the way your body feels when you drink a truly rehydrating beverage. How does this feeling differ from the effects you feel when you drink a caffeinated beverage instead?

- **On: Give H_2O a Chance**

  1. Over the course of the next week or so, try to consciously work through the tips on retraining your taste buds to appreciate water as a beverage. Over the course of this period, make a note of how your beverage preferences may be changing.

- **On: Tuning into Thirst**

  1. Discuss the steps that you can take to become a better "thirst sensor"?

  2. What happens if you try to fill up on liquids before a meal? Why might this be a poor technique for curbing your appetite?

  3. You have already learned that diet drinks are poor thirst-quenchers. Discuss some of the other ways that they help confuse your body's thirst and hunger signals? In your discussion, consider how the sugar and other additives may influence your taste preferences.

  4. The marketing hype about diet drinks gives many people the illusion that these beverages can somehow, miraculously, offset poor eating habits. Discuss some examples of this, drawing from advertising or from your own observations.

- **On: Signs of Dehydration**

  1. Discuss the symptoms of dehydration and how they can have a negative impact upon your health, physical comfort, and feelings of well-being. What steps can you take to avoid these impacts?

The Guided Journal

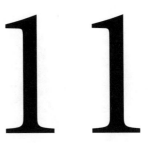

Why Keep a Journal?
Ready, Set . . . Journal!
A Peek into a Real Journal

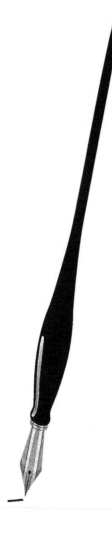

I s your energy low? Does it seem like you are eating automatically or compulsively when you feel down or discouraged? Do monthly variations in your mood, eating, or energy patterns have you confused?

If you answered "yes" to any of these questions, then the seven-day guided journal presented in this chapter can help. The simple act of writing down how you feel and what you eat throughout the day will reward you with a wealth of information that will help you understand—and eventually solve—your eating dilemmas. The reason this journal works is because it uncovers your unique issues. Instead of following a one-size-fits-all plan, you can tailor your strategy to your own lifestyle and needs.

Why Keep a Journal?

An ongoing journal that chronicles your days while specifically noting your eating and lifestyle behavior serves a number of worthwhile purposes. For example, keeping a journal:

- Provides a realistic assessment of your eating patterns and habits.
- Makes you more aware of your daily activity levels.
- Helps you define your hunger and fullness points.
- Identifies your emotional reasons for eating (for instance, eating when you're bored, stressed, or upset).
- Helps you uncover "diet thinking" (as in journal entries like "I ate 'bad' foods today," or "After eating that I wanted to go on a diet").
- Tracks your successes by revealing your change in attitude over time.
- Provides an outlet for feelings, both positive and negative.

Keep in mind that it's really a diary or journal—*not* just a food record. You enter more than just a list of the foods you eat—you also write down your feelings, your activities, and your observations about life.

Keeping a journal is harder than it looks. You have to build some special time into your day when you can reflect on how you're feeling, get in touch with those feelings and your responses to them, and then find the courage to commit those feelings and actions to paper. But the experience is very satisfying and rewarding. And when you're done, you can applaud yourself for completing something difficult!

The process of pausing, reflecting, and writing will slow you down just enough to make some very interesting self-discoveries. These discoveries will help you to be more aware of your daily life, and that awareness will help you improve your method of coping. You'll begin to recognize patterns: how you respond to crises, how you deal with feelings, how you view food, and how your body speaks to you through hunger and thirst cues (cravings) and exhaustion.

Ready, Set . . . Journal!

Keeping a journal is generally a three step process. Step one is preparing a written snapshot of your current lifestyle. Step two is keeping your seven-day food record. The process of keeping the food journal will empower your self-awareness. It will be as unique as you are. Step three is the interpretation stage—an opportunity for you to reflect upon and evaluate what your eating and activity habits are trying to tell you. Here are the ground rules for effectively taking these three steps:

1. *The Written Portrait.* Spend some time reflecting on your present lifestyle, and then create a written portrait of yourself. This description should include your family situation, your work and daily routine, your past food or weight experiences, your approach and attitude to fitness and activity, and any self-discovery findings that are important to you. You'll probably write about two pages. You're tuning in.

2. *The Event, Food, and Feeling Record.* For seven days, record your daily eating, drinking and activity habits, along with your emotional and physical feelings before and after food and activity.

3. *Interpretation.* Your next step is to pinpoint some area where you can make a small improvement and work on that for awhile. In my experience, it helps to share your new step towards change with a trusted, supportive person or a group. If you keep it to yourself you can easily feel overwhelmed, or indulge in procrastination. But if you share your new decision with someone in your support circle who can check in with you and show interest in your progress, your chances of sustained change are increased. If you have no support network in place yet, you can contact HUGS International, Inc.— we offer a journal analysis service (contact information is included at the end of this book).

While keeping your journal, continue your typical eating and activity patterns at first. You need to be careful not to consciously make changes in your present patterns simply because you are writing them down. Only an accurate reflection of what's been going on in your life will allow you to figure out what needs fixing and then to fix it.

Write down everything you eat and drink. You don't have to record exact quantities of food, just a general description. It is important to note each time you eat or drink. At the same time, tune into how you were feeling before and after each time you eat. Write these feelings down in the second and fourth column of the table.

As with your eating record, you'll want to keep a record of your daily activities for one week. Make a note of such events as taking a walk, watching TV, or going out to eat, and be sure to record any emotional event—such as having a fight with your mate—as well. Most important, keep your focus on how you feel and on your hunger and fullness, and do not get too obsessed with food quantities or in judging the types of food you eat in this part.

Instead of looking at the diary as a way to berate yourself for not eating "perfectly," consider it simply as a way to discover how deeply you're in the grip of the diet mentality. You'll soon see where diet thinking still has some hold on your thoughts. For instance, you'll discover that you're reluctant to write down certain foods because you consider them to be "bad." But that's an important point of the journal—to give you an opportunity to identify the areas where diet thinking still has a grip on you.

A Peek Into a Real Journal

It's always easier to get started in a new activity like journaling if you can see how other people have done it. Sandra Olafson, a HUGS participant who went the extra mile and had her journal analyzed by me, has graciously agreed to share her own journaling experience in hopes that it will inspire you to try it, too.

Before Sandra heard about the HUGS program (in an article in the July 1999 issue of the Canadian women's magazine, *Chatelaine*) she had been through a slew of weight-loss programs, including Weight Watchers, Nutri-System, and TOPS. Now she was ready for a new approach. There were no HUGS programs in her area so she decided to join our HUGS at Home program for support while she got herself in order and improved her health—in other words, while she learned more about getting off the diet rollercoaster.

Since she had no local support network, Sandra decided to use the HUGS Journal Analysis Service. Upon filling out her journal, she shipped it off to me and in return I provided her with a customized report and commentary that provided her with a detailed analysis of why she had been experiencing ups and downs, along with tips and suggestions on keeping her lifestyle patterns focused on health and energy. She was affirmed in areas where she was already on track and guided through areas that could be improved. The emphasis was on slow and gradual changes that will evolve into lifetime habits.

Sandra hopes that as you work through her journaling experience you will pick up on patterns that may help you interpret your own journal analysis. Look for areas in which you might identify with Sandra's patterns. Find areas that you might need to work on. This process will help you understand what journaling is all about. And as you identify unhealthy patterns in your own lifestyle, you'll be able to go back through this book to find the specific chapters that address the issues that concern you.

Sandra's Written Portrait: "I should have been born a bear"

I'm 43 and quite tired of the diet rollercoaster. I've been programmed in since about age 15. I've been every size from 5–6 to present 14, 16, 18. I'm a registered nurse and work shift work at the local hospital on the medical-surgical ward. I'm married to a commercial pilot who is away from home a lot and who is naturally thin and a chocoholic. We have three active children, all teenagers, Stefan 19, Scott 17, Pam 14, and all, so far, naturally thin.

I'm a "doer," mostly for others, and I usually ignore my own needs. I'm also a worrier, so I do "stress" eat. I could control my weight until after having had Pam. After her birth I developed Hashimoto's thyroiditis, leaving me hypothyroid, and losing weight was much more difficult. We lived overseas for four years from 1985–1989. I was thin then because I did not work outside the home and instead worked out two hours or more each day swimming, biking, walking, and at the gym. Since moving back to Canada and northwestern Ontario and returning to the workforce I have steadily climbed the scales going from 135 lbs. to my present 174 lbs. in the last ten years. When I ignore dieting and eat properly I can lose one to two pounds per week. This lasts one to two weeks. With my mid-cycle PMS all is lost with the cravings. I seem to have gotten this somewhat under control in the last two months with eating every three hours and taking supplemental calcium, magnesium, vitamin B complex, E, and C which seem to have helped me control some of the stressful (PMS) eating that I seem to go through from Day 14–28 of my cycle.

I know that I must put more activity in my day and plan ahead to eat well, but just don't or can't seem to organize that for a consecutive 30 or more days. Also winter is bad. I'm sure I suffer from seasonal affective disorder because I always feel much better from May to October, then awful from October to May needing twice as much sleep and food especially comfort carbohydrates. I awake at dawn and go to bed one to two hours after dark, great in summer but winter I'm pretty pathetic. I should have been born a bear.

I'm caffeine intolerant and alcohol doesn't do much for me so I pretty much avoid these. I'm 5'4" (probably shrunk since last measuring). I carry my weight in the middle of my torso, a definite risk. So that's why I would like to shape up, eat better, feel more vigorous each day, and like myself 365 days, not just on my good days. That is why I have joined HUGS.

Sandra's Written Portrait: My Reaction

Sandra, congratulations on taking the first step to getting off the diet rollercoaster. You have certainly identified some of the problem areas that keep you from a diet-free lifestyle and it sounds like you are prepared to do something about it. The first step is awareness and the next step is action. Let's talk about some action steps.

1. You are a "doer" for others and ignore your own needs. This can lead to feelings of resentment, which are totally natural, but which can lead to eating for comfort. You absolutely need to put aside time for yourself and protect this time for you and you alone. Be firm, be

assertive, state your needs to your family and why. This will only come back to them in the sense that they will learn some life skills of responsibility and you will have more enjoyable time with them; you will be rejuvenated.

2. You are a worrier, and you turn to food while worrying. Next time you catch yourself eating while worrying, put in that "pause" as you see yourself reaching for the food. Ask yourself these questions:

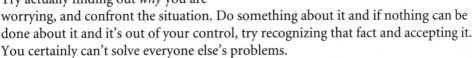

    • Does eating help the worries?
    • Do you actually taste your food when you are eating for this reason?

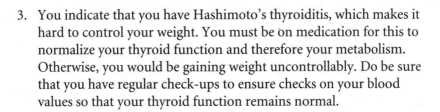

If the answer to the two questions is no, then what's the point? Why eat? It's simply a waste of food, time, and calories. Try actually finding out *why* you are worrying, and confront the situation. Do something about it and if nothing can be done about it and it's out of your control, try recognizing that fact and accepting it. You certainly can't solve everyone else's problems.

3. You indicate that you have Hashimoto's thyroiditis, which makes it hard to control your weight. You must be on medication for this to normalize your thyroid function and therefore your metabolism. Otherwise, you would be gaining weight uncontrollably. Do be sure that you have regular check-ups to ensure checks on your blood values so that your thyroid function remains normal.

As an aside, I had hyperthyroidism, which is very hard to regulate with medication, and so I needed to take the radioactive iodine, which left me hypothyroid. The upside to all of this is that hypothyroidism is much more easily regulated with the replacement hormone that has no side effects. So if some reason, you are not on medication, do ensure that you check with your doctor.

4. You hit upon a change in your life—less physical activity—and being active is really key for health and weight stabilization.

And it sounds like your time overseas allowed you to enjoy physical activity for fun and the other health benefits kicked in.

5. Coming home to Canada perhaps resulted in a heavier workload as you returned to the workforce, had less free time, and more stress. And then with taking care of everyone else's needs on top of that, where is the time for you? Your food can easily become your companion, and unconscious eating can result—eating when you are worrying, eating when you are in a hurry, grabbing food, instead of paying attention to tastes, foods, flavors, and aromas. You may be missing out on the true experience of tasting and savoring your food and you're certainly eating for other reasons than physical hunger. Physical activity, if you give it a try, should have the greatest impact in helping alleviate PMS. The endorphins, that feel-good chemical that kicks in, will do wonders in balancing out those hormonal cravings.

6. It may be hard for you to take care of yourself for longer than a month at a time because your life may just be too full. Do you schedule in padded time for those unexpected emergencies or are you always in a hurry, flying out the door? It's quite normal for many people to feel better and have more energy with more daylight hours. For many women when there is a season change, a drain of energy occurs. Don't fight it; go with it; do what you need to do to help counterbalance the lack of energy. Rest more, build in more "time out" for yourself, and include the word "no" in your vocabulary more often.

You have recognized that this is a pattern from October to May and so adjust your activities accordingly. Yes, it's about acceptance again. Some things we just can't change. And recognizing your age, soon you will begin to feel the symptoms of menopause. To prepare for this, be careful of the multitasking. Memory lapses may occur and it's easier if you have adjusted to doing one thing at a time instead of trying to do a bunch of things at the same time and then wondering why you have such a hard time keeping organized. Maybe you are simply trying to do too much. Refer to the last chapter in *You Count, Calories Don't* on menopause—it will prepare you for the near future.

Remember that in the past, you haven't failed; the diets failed *you*. This is an important affirmation to repeat to yourself if you ever have a doubt and think that you had failures in the past. The diet industry has such a clever way of marketing that they get people to believe that the diet worked and if they go "off" the diet, that they don't have enough willpower and they failed. Did you ever wonder why the diet industry is a billion-dollar business? Yes, that's right; it's because it is a really good *repeat* business, where people go on and off the diet for the rest of their lives.

You've made super progress by including more fluids (especially water with your meals), eating regularly, and not avoiding food when hungry. Transfer this new skill to other areas of your life and don't avoid your other life needs. Listening to your body's needs for food, rest, and water is so important. This is a great start. You will want to gradually work in more rehydrating fluids into your day as you note that you may still be far from the recommended 8–10 glasses per day of rehydrating fluid intake (especially water). Take it one step at a time; think of ways to work in activity that will work for you and then begin gradually doing it. Be careful not to apply the diet thinking and do-it-all-at-once-then-nothing-at-all syndrome. (About your PMS, check pages 41 and 42 in *You Count, Calories Don't* for some guidance.)

Sandra's Event, Food, and Feeling Record

DAY 1			
Time range and Activity	Feelings before eating	Food	Feelings after eating
7:30–8:00 a.m.: Making, eating breakfast	hungry, wanting to start day off well	1 large egg, 2 slices flax bread, butter, fieldberry jam, orange	food tasted good, satisfied. *Ate for physical comfort.*
8:00–10:00 a.m.: reading, running around, making stew, etc., copying tape for later walking.	quiet	None	bit disorganized
11:45 a.m.: washing floor	starting of hunger, stomach feels empty, know I'm going out for lunch at 12:30, don't want to be ravenous when I order.	1 glass soya milk and water	satisfied, *probably hunger is real, but I sure was thirsty too.*

Time range and activity	Feelings before eating	Food	Feelings after eating
12:30 p.m.	happy to be with friends for lunch.	creamy turkey soup, 1/2 chicken salad on a bun, Earl Grey tea	ate till I was full, took breaks to talk about friends' lives, new happenings, focus on eating. *I did well, found it difficult to really taste each bite and concentrate on food when I was listening and talking.*
3:30–11:30 p.m.: work shift evenings	this 3–4 p.m. time always my low time; always feel I need a snack to get me through to supper	hot chocolate, chocolate cake	
6:00 p.m.: supper break, not too hungry	blood sugars when checked are always in low end	1/2 portion stew partridge, cheese, biscuit, raspberry jam, milk, tea	cheese biscuit wasn't that great, *should have gone for bread, otherwise satisfied*
8:30 p.m.: coffee break	busy evening, not sure if eating out of comfort	2 digestive cookies, tea	satisfied, *ready to start heavy evening routine round at work*
12:00 midnight	hungry	small bowl cereal, milk	

Day 1, My Comments

Sandra, this sounds like a nice day, and you are certainly tuning in to your feelings and paying attention to the food you eat. Be careful, though, not to eat when you think you "should" eat (recollections of dieting, perhaps) and eat when your body says it's *time* to eat. What I mean by this is that feeling hungry around 11:45 a.m. after eating breakfast at 7:30–8 a.m. is totally normal and expected. If you anticipate having a later lunch, plugging in a snack works well—as you did with the soya milk (which is more substantial a beverage than water or juice).

You had hearty bread (flax bread) for breakfast with butter and jam along with the egg as the protein source, which held you over well through the next 4-hour stretch. And if you are finding that 3–4 p.m. is the time you generally need a snack, don't fight it; go for it. That snack time might be pushed up on days that you eat lunch later. Snacks are great for dampening your hunger so that at mealtime you come to the table pleasantly hungry, rather than ravenous.

You are really getting on to this! One more thing . . . I note that you checked your blood sugar at 6 p.m. and it was on the low end. I haven't noted that you have diabetes; are you just checking to see if your body's hunger level coincides with what the numbers say about blood sugar level? This certainly will help you tune in better. If you weren't too hungry by 6 p.m., 5 hours after lunch and 2 hours after your snack, then maybe your snack might have been too much. Careful not to skimp on your meals. You are tuning in to what you really like though, and recognizing that the cheese biscuit may not have been as satisfying as the bread. Sometimes things look better than they actually taste and may not do the job of filling us up and satisfying us as well.

DAY 2			
Time range and activity	Feelings before eating	Food	Feelings after eating
All day	Feel blah today, tired, bloated, no energy		
9:30 a.m.		egg, 2 slices flax bread, jam, orange, tea with milk	*not much change in energy level, draggy*
11:00 a.m.	Decided to cook, don't feel much like anything else	1/2 cup apple crisp with 1/4 cup plain yogurt, 4 prunes, tea with milk	*still blah*

Time range and activity	Feelings before eating	Food	Feelings after eating
1:00 p.m.	It's lunch time, should eat something, pizza in fridge	2 small slices pepperoni cheese pizza eaten out, 4 oz. V8 juice	quite salty, *wondering if this was the best choice,* drank 1–2 glasses water, energy up a little
5:00 p.m.	hungry, no one home for supper so decided on leftovers again	2 small slices pizza, milk 16 oz., apple	
7:00 p.m.	comfort food cravings	Gingerbread cookie dough and cookies, tea with milk	*enjoyed first few bites and then ate a few more than I needed, beat and guilty*

Day 2, My Comments

You didn't feel well today and made food adjustments accordingly. You took the hassle out of meal preparation by going with leftovers, just allowed yourself to feel "blah," and went with the feeling. Good for you! It's totally normal not to feel good all the time.

You were right on target by minimizing your expectations of yourself. And at supper you may have eaten a few more cookies than you wanted (note you used the word "needed"—watch out for diet thinking) and you felt guilty. Yet your reaction to the guilt has improved. Think back to what used to happen when there was guilt . . . you probably thought one of two things:

1. "I blew the diet anyway, so I might as well binge on some more cookies"; or

2. "I'll go into diet mode the next day to compensate for the extra cookies." But this only leads to bingeing down the road, and the starve-binge cycle—that is, the on again/off again dieting—would resume. Sandra, you licked this one! Congratulations!

DAY 3			
Time range and activity	**Feelings before eating**	**Food**	**Feelings after eating**
9:00 a.m.	awake refreshed	2 slices flax bread, jam, egg, orange	start day with good breakfast, happy, *content with my choice, enjoyed and tasted*
12:30–1:00 p.m., walk with dog	beautiful sunshine day, cool, uplifted		
1:30–2:00 p.m.	craving for a hot dog, also hungry after walking	small bowl baked beans, hot dog (low fat, bun and condiments, large skim milk, tea with milk	hungry prior, *enjoyed eating and savoring, spending lunch with family,* satisfied with amounts eaten
3:05–5:00 p.m. walk	refreshed, uplifted, and a bit tired	water	rehydrated
4:30–4:45 p.m.		1 slice banana bread, 1 tsp. peanut butter, apple	hungry, supper still 1 hour away, feel good selection, ate it slowly, enjoyed flavors, satisfied following, content to wait for supper
5:30–5:45 p.m.		partridge stew, thick slice dill bread, small bowl caramel light ice milk and apple crisp	satisfied, ate, tasted, enjoyed
6:30–8:00 p.m.		tea with milk	watching TV with husband eating peanuts *feel good that I averted peanuts*

Time range and activity	Feelings before eating	Food	Feelings after eating
8:00 p.m.	hungry	10 oz. soya milk, Harvest Crunch cereal, 1/3 cup	

Day 3, My Comments

Wow! Are you ever tuned in here! It sounds like that "taking it easy" day 2 allowed you the time to do what you needed to help your body regenerate. It totally makes sense that you might have felt blah or tired on day 2 after a late work night on day 1. You did what it took to allow your body to rest, heal, and regenerate—and you ended up with a great day 3. You had nice walks, enjoyed the process of eating and savoring your food, and fueled your body when it was hungry. And bravo! You didn't eat the peanuts while watching TV just because your husband was eating them, because you didn't want them, you were not hungry. You licked the automatic eating!

DAY 4			
Time range and activity	Feelings before eating	Food	Feelings after eating
9:30–10:00 a.m.: breakfast	hungry	oatmeal, dried cranberries, 1 tsp. flax, 1 cup skim milk, 1/2 cup 1 percent milk	hunger relief, ate slow, savored, enjoyed
10:00–10:30 a.m.: light exercise	waken my body and mind to start day		relaxed and stretched out
12:00 noon	hungry, thirsty	egg salad sandwich on French bread, soya milk, apple, tea	
12:45–1:10p.m.: walk	uplifted, refreshed		

Time range and activity	Feelings before eating	Food	Feelings after eating
1:15–3:30 p.m.: was out shopping		1 glass Chai tea, 1 soft gingerbread cookie	bit thirsty, hungry
5:00 p.m.: Icing Christmas cakes		almond paste, few bites	
7:00–8:00 p.m.: Christian Women's Club Dinner	enjoy being out	turkey with gravy, stuffing, carrots, salad, cranberries, chocolate mousse desert, tea	enjoying tasting dinner and tried to slow down my eating, *probably could have stopped at two tastes of dessert* and felt quite full following
9:30 p.m.		6 oz. soya milk with evening pills	

Day 4, My Comments

Another nice day awaited you. Another accomplishment . . . you ate regularly and didn't succumb to the "I'm going out for dinner so I'm going to save up for it and not eat all day." This allowed you to come to the supper table and eat more slowly, savoring every bite instead of gulping your food down. It sounds like you felt that you ate more dessert than you "needed," which is diet thinking. This experience of feeling quite full doesn't sound like you overate; there is a definite difference between "quite full" and stuffed.

DAYS 5			
Time range and activity	Feelings before eating	Food	Feelings after eating
9:00 a.m.		1 slice French toast, milk, maple syrup	

Time range and activity	Feelings before eating	Food	Feelings after eating
10:00 a.m. to 12 noon: housecleaning			
12:00–1:00 p.m.: lunch at noon with my sister	hungry	tomato with rice soup, 1/2 salmon sandwich, pickles, milk, tea with milk	satisfied, not stuffed
1:00–3:00 p.m.: housecleaning			
3:30–4:00 p.m.: snack		tea with milk, slice of banana bread with peanut butter, banana	satisfied
5:00–5:30 p.m.: supper		small serving lasagna, 2 slices garlic toast, apple	satisfied but *wondered if I should have made a salad too?*
6:45 p.m.	wanted a little something sweet	tea with milk, small bowl chocolate ice milk	
9:00 p.m.	hungry? PMS craving	popcorn with pretzel mix (3 cups)	wanted something crunchy, bit salty but still healthy

Day 5, My Comments

Yes, you've got it! You ate lunch and noted that it made you feel satisfied, not stuffed. You sound tuned into feelings of satiety, how full you are. For supper, you had lasagna and two slices of garlic toast and an apple. You wondered if you "should" have made a salad too. Definitely, a salad with pasta dish rounds out the meal and includes more of the vegetable component. Having garlic toast adds more of the starch and carbohydrate along with fat. However, if this is part of your tradition of eating pasta, then perhaps you could compromise with one slice less garlic toast but add a salad.

And you seem to be tuned into what you want—something sweet; something crunchy, something salty—and you are satisfying your PMS cravings accordingly. To be specific, your small bowl of chocolate ice milk satisfied your sweet craving, while the popcorn with pretzel mix took care of the crunchy-salty craving—and in a healthy way!

DAY 6			
Time range and activity	**Feelings before eating**	**Food**	**Feelings after eating**
10:00–10:45 a.m.: breakfast	hungry for something nutritious, satisfying	1 scrambled egg, 3 mini potatoes, 1 tbsp. bacon bits, large glass orange juice, tea with milk	light-hearted, happy, contented, full. *I'm feeling really good about myself and food choices, especially during this PMS time as this is usually my worst time*
1:30–1:45 p.m.: lunch	hungry	small plate spaghetti with sauce, 1 slice cheese garlic bread, V8 juice, tomato	ate a little fast, *didn't concentrate as much as I should have* but realized at times and stopped and tried to get myself back on track
2:00–4:00 p.m.: laundry			
6:30–7:00 p.m.: dinner	family made supper for me	4 breaded chicken fingers, mashed potatoes, raw carrots with dill dip, pickles, cranberry jelly	
7:00–9:00 p.m.: housework			
9:00–11:00 p.m. watch TV			

Day 6, My Comments

Wow! You are into PMS time and are feeling good about your choices—and you certainly *deserve* to feel that way. Recognizing your cravings, working with them, and trying to eat healthier minimizes the blood-sugar swings that can come during this time and lead to more cravings. Reread part on PMS in chapter 1 of *You Count, Calories Don't*. And this turned out to be another nice day; even the family made supper for you. What a treat!

DAY 7			
Time range and activity	**Feelings before eating**	**Food**	**Feelings after eating**
7:00 a.m.: ready for work	worked 12 hour day, busy steady on feet most of day except breaks	soya milk	need something to start the day that's nutritious but light
10:00 a.m.	hungry	oatmeal, cranberries, flax, skim milk, tea with 2 percent creamers	enjoyed, satisfied
1:00 p.m.	sounded good	Chinese special cafeteria, 4 chicken balls, 4 pineapple chicken, 4 spareribs, oriental vegetables, egg roll, sweet and sour sauce, tea	didn't taste as good as I thought it would but I still ate it all. *Should have been more selective*
3:30 p.m.	mid afternoon energy slump	popcorn, pretzel mix, 2 cups, water	enjoyed, savored, satisfied
6:00 p.m.	hungry	tuna sandwich, pea pods, carrots, tomato, V8 juice	really enjoyed this meal, really tasting my food well
7:30–9:00 p.m.: shopping	not too hungry when I came home but pizza was out	2 slices Deluxe Kraft frozen pizza	enjoyed but probably could have skipped these calories

Time range and activity	Feelings before eating	Food	Feelings after eating
11:00 p.m.	thirsty, needed something to take night vitamins	soya milk	

Day 7, My Comments

This is a super busy 12-hour work day for you. It's nice that you had some previous nice days to prepare for the intensity of this day! It helps to keep your balance. You did well! Even though you may have eaten everything on your plate at the Chinese special cafeteria lunch, you recognized that perhaps you could be more selective. This awareness will help you next time around. In other words, you need not eat it just because it's there; eat it because you want it, like it, and are hungry for it.

The comment of "It didn't taste as good as I thought but I still ate it all" may mean that you were hungry or that you could have left some on your plate (the less favorites) if you were satisfied and full. For supper though, you recognized this fact, and were sure tuned into tasting your food and enjoying your sandwich, veggies, and V-8 juice.

Sandra, you should be pleased at your progress! At this point, you are close to finishing the program and well past the usual two weeks–1 month span you usually last on traditional diets. In fact, you were past this point when you sent me the journal. Enjoy how good this can make you feel. Realize that from time to time your life may be out of balance; use the quiet times as an opportunity to get tuned back in. Enjoy!

Taking It Deeper

This time let's Take It Deeper in a way that's different from earlier chapters—after all, in one way you're Taking It Deeper throughout the chapter by starting a journal, right? In this section, though, try your hand at your own analysis of Sandra's journal. Where would you add to or expand upon my own analysis? While you're trying this exercise, keep the following questions, keyed to the individual days, in mind:

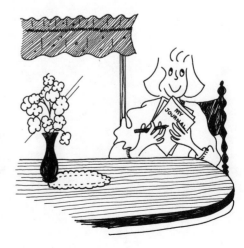

- Day 1: What demonstrates that Sandra is learning to eat when pleasantly hungry and not wait till she is ravenous? What is Sandra learning about satisfying foods in her experimenting with foods?

- Day 2: What happens if you allow yourself to feel guilty after eating too much? What happens if you take time out and slow down when you don't feel good?

- Day 3: How did Sandra's choice to "go with" her blah feelings on Day 2 affect her next day's experience? How did she avoid automatic eating?

- Day 4: How did Sandra handle eating out? Discuss her experience. How is Sandra using a gradual process of tailoring her tastes to alter her eating habits?

- Day 5: How was Sandra able to tune into her feelings of hunger and fullness? How was Sandra tuned into what types of food she wanted? Answer Sandra's question on adding a salad to lasagna meal.

- Day 6: Why was Sandra able to go through this PMS time smoothly? Review her 5 previous days' experiences for clues to her success on this 6th day.

- Day 7: How did Sandra prepare for her long, 12-hour work day? How would you guide Sandra in eating until satisfied when eating out? Sandra recognized that she could have been more selective. Do you have any suggestions for her?

Tailoring Your Tastes 12

Five Fundamentals
Enjoyable Eating
Taste Fundamental #1
    The big decision
    Snack saviors
Taste Fundamental #2
    Fear of fat
    Is your diet too low in fat?
    Enjoying the taste of health
    Guide to tailoring your tastes
Taste Fundamental #3
    Bring your children into the experiment
Taste Fundamental #4
Tailoring Your Tastes—In Action!
Recipe Concepts
    The recipe makeover
    Sunshine muffins

What's your biggest barrier to healthier eating? If you're like many people, it's taste. North American taste buds have been brought up on fast foods, mediocre vegetables and fruits, and a culinary tradition that uses fat to make things tasty. No wonder a leaner, more vegetable-rich diet seems like a prison sentence. But Japanese taste buds prefer sushi, miso soup, and other leaner foods. Mediterranean taste buds appreciate both an olive-oil and cheese-rich lasagna or moussaka as well as a simple dessert of in-season, fabulous watermelons or grapes.

The point: we humans can tailor our tastes to any type of eating. We're not permanently programmed to prefer fries over carrots, Ben and Jerry's Chubby Hubby over sorbet. What's not so easy—and the downfall of many a valiant effort to healthy-up our eating—is overnight radical change.

In this chapter, I'm going to show you how to slowly and comfortably tailor your tastes towards healthier eating. The goal of tailoring your tastes is to acquire the tools to help you gradually move your taste preferences toward foods that are lower in fat, sugar, and salt and higher in fiber. You'll shift from higher-fat to lower-fat eating, and from the occasional vegetable and fruit to a diet rich in these foods. You'll keep choosing healthful foods because you *want to* rather than because you have to.

And if you'd like to go further in-depth on this issue, check out the *Tailoring Your Tastes* cookbook, which you can order through my HUGS web site.

Five Fundamentals

Retraining your taste buds to a new way of eating is not as hard as you might think. But as with learning any new way of doing things, there are some things you can do to make the change easier. I've come up with five keys to successfully tailoring your tastes—and you've already mastered one of them! Yes, that's right—back in Chapter 10, when you learned how to tune into your body's hunger and thirst signals, you were learning the first step toward successfully tailoring your taste buds. Now it's time to learn about the other four keys to success.

1. *Take Your Time.* Tastes take a lifetime to develop, and can't be changed quickly. But gradual doesn't mean rigidly moving from an original version of a food to a low-fat version. How regimented it would be to have to follow such a schedule—this week the original, next week a lower-fat version, and the lowest-fat type in the week after *that*! Some people just aren't ready to make the change on that kind of schedule.

Instead, gradual change means eating at the level you are comfortable with, and *staying* there until you fully appreciate the tastes and textures of this variation. Only then do you make the next adjustment. This may take three months, six months—or even more. Maybe you won't ever get to a *really* low-fat, low-sugar, high-fiber level . . . but that's okay. Going gradual is a progression along a constantly improving nutrition profile—at your own pace.

2. *Respect Your Tastes.* "Head knowledge" about healthy foods doesn't translate into the desire to eat them. It's a matter of very individual choice. Your tastes are unique and are quite likely different even from others in your family. Find out how to respect and work with your tastes. For many of you, this probably involves overcoming a fear of fat that you've learned over a lifetime. Just remember that severely cutting back fat usually means cutting back on the tastes you grew up with—and that's clearly *not* respecting your taste preferences.

3. *Be willing to experiment.* You'll have a lot more fun, and wind up with a more nutritious diet, if you're willing to experiment. This means not only trying new foods or new food combinations, but also trying out new proportions of the different types of foods—in particular, the balance of carbohydrates to proteins you include in a meal. Gradually shift the food on your plate to include more carbs (2/3 to 3/4) and less protein (1/3 to 1/4). Use the "divided plate" image to remind you how this works. You'll probably have to do a little experimenting to find out just what is the most satisfying proportion for your own, personal nutritional needs. Remember, this can't happen overnight—finding new satisfying ways of eating requires patience.

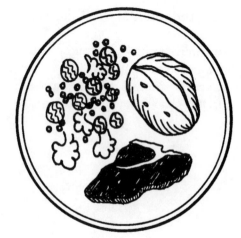

4. *Learn a few culinary tricks of the trade.* Did you know that you can substitute half-and-half or evaporated milk for cream and still wind up with a satisfyingly creamy fish chowder? Or, that no one will notice that your thick,

delicious cheese sauce was based on flour and one percent milk instead of whole milk or cream? It's worth your while to learn a few ways to lower the fat or up the fiber and nutrients in your food while retaining the taste and satisfying "mouth feel" of your favorite dishes.

Learning new cooking skills and tricks can make a big difference in successfully changing your food preferences. Changing minor details in preparation—such as a little spritz of lemon here, a dash of olive oil or fresh basil there—can change your mind about a vegetable or bean dish you never really cared for in the past. When I expand on this taste fundamental later on in the chapter, I'll share with you some of the techniques that have been particularly valuable to me.

Enjoyable eating

- Take satisfying portions; you can always have seconds if you are still hungry.
- Eat slowly so that you taste, savor and enjoy each mouthful. Focus on the food you are eating; you'll feel satisfied with less.
- Put a pause into your meal; tell an interesting story. Stop eating when you are satisfied; you don't have to clean your plate.
- If the menu includes a particular favorite, be sure to have a satisfactory amount. If necessary, balance it out by having a little less of the less interesting foods. Remember, denying yourself puts you smack dab back into the diet mentality.

Taste Fundamental #1: Take Your Time

When you're working to retrain your taste buds, you've got a choice: you can try to get it done in one "Big Jump" or you can opt for the "Smooth Slide" into a new way of eating. Obviously, I favor the smooth slide—a gradual change is far more likely to be a lasting change. If you contrast the two approaches you can easily see why.

The big decision: I've decided that the whole family is going to move toward healthier eating.

	THE BIG JUMP	THE SMOOTH SLIDE
First action on making the decision	Brace Yourself: Quickly eat all your favorite foods because you know they won't be part of your diet tomorrow.	Feel Good About Yourself: Feel good that you've made the conscious decision to start making slow changes that will reflect a healthier lifestyle.
First shopping trip for healthy food	Stock up on foods that say "light," "low-fat," or "diet" on the labels, regardless of whether you enjoy them. For example, your family likes whole milk, but you buy skim instead.	Stock up on a wide variety of foods that you and your family enjoy, paying more attention to moving toward more carb-rich foods and fewer high-protein foods. Buy a few herbs to enhance the flavors of your meals. You pick up some two-percent milk knowing that if your family doesn't care for it right away you can mix it half and half with whole milk until they learn to like the lighter mouth feel.
Feelings of the cook after 1 week	Frustrated and overwhelmed. Food is drier than the family enjoys. Still, cook has strong resolve to keep trying, even if the rest of the family isn't enthusiastic.	Encouraged by how easy it has been so far to make small changes at mealtimes. Family seems to enjoy the new cooking techniques and have adjusted to the new balance of carbs and proteins. Cook is pleasantly surprised that family hasn't complained.

	THE BIG JUMP	THE SMOOTH SLIDE
		Notices that the new way of cooking results in foods with a nicer color and texture, and are as flavorful as foods cooked the "old" way.
Reactions of family after 1 week	Concerned that food will never be "tasty" anymore. Tired of the new, chewier and drier tastes and textures at mealtimes. Longing for last week's menu. Growing proficient at slipping food to grateful canine under the table. Wishing the budget allowed more order-in or eat-out foods for next week. Snacking and eating away from home as often as possible.	Surprised that they still get to eat the foods they love! Notice that their foods have more color, more interesting textures, and as much if not more flavor than before. Feel more energized after a meal, instead of tired and overfull.
Feelings of cook at 1 month	Almost ready to give up because nobody is enjoying the food at mealtimes. Disappointed and feeling deprived. Missing the old way of cooking and missing all the foods that have been given up. Wishing that the new way of cooking wasn't such an overwhelming chore. Starting to sneak "old favorites" more and more frequently.	Excited that the process is still so enjoyable. Not even *thinking* about quitting. Having more and more fun experimenting with old and new recipes and feeling pleased with the results, flavors, and textures.

	THE BIG JUMP	THE SMOOTH SLIDE
Reactions of family at 1 month	Ready to move in with the neighbors during mealtimes. Wishing the "health kick" at the house would end. Eating out or ordering in as often as possible and when eating the foods they like, really eating *lots*. Snacking and sneaking foods more and more often.	Still enjoying the food that's on the table. Asking for certain new favorites more often: "When are you going to make that great bread again?" Noticing that they aren't hungry between meals as often as they used to be.
Reaction of family and cook at 3 months	Disillusioned with the "health movement." Disappointed and feeling a little guilty, they give up and return to the old ways of eating and cooking. Some of the family actually rejoice at the chance to go back to eating what they love!	Everybody feels good about themselves and the new way of eating and preparing foods. Energized by their success, the whole family wants to keep up the effort to develop healthier eating habits. As an experiment, they may even try a food favorite from the old days and are surprised and pleased to discover that they actually have come to like the new foods better!

Clearly, the gradual approach is the way to go! And always keep in mind, that if a change doesn't feel right, you can slow down your process toward healthier eating until you're more comfortable with it. Recognize that *any* change is progress, and that striving for a particular endpoint is falling back into the diet thinking. Make improved health your goal. And while you're experimenting with new foods and new ways to prepare them, tailor your tastes by taking the time to appreciate the subtle differences in taste, texture, and mouth-feel of healthier foods. If they are not becoming choices you make because you prefer and enjoy them, then you are returning to the diet mentality.

Snack saviors

If you need a snack, eat it. Otherwise, you will be so hungry by the next meal that you'll wolf down your food without really savoring it. Eat regularly, letting your physical hunger and appetite be your guide. Try introducing more carbohydrates such as whole grain bread, lower fat muffins, yogurt, and fruit.

Do not restrict yourself to salads alone—while they may fill you up temporarily, they don't have much substance and may lead to bingeing later on. And don't be fooled into thinking salads are always light; a large Caesar salad can be twice as fat-laden as a roast beef sandwich. The roast beef, or turkey or other meat-based sandwich, on the other hand, will hold you over a lot longer and leave you feeling more satisfied. Therefore, the point is to focus more on the satisfaction, taste, and "holdover power" of foods and meals, rather than the content of fat and calories.

Taste Fundamental #2: Respect Your Tastes

Your tastes may have evolved from the prevailing culture, or from growing up with an ethnic cuisine, such as Mexican, Arabic, or Asian. There are healthful foods in all cuisines, and there are ways of making some of the dishes in every cuisine more healthful. Be proud of your "taste heritage" and find out how to use it to improve your eating.

That's one part of respecting your tastes. The other part is to stop denying yourself foods and tastes you love out of a fear that they're unhealthy. That's usually a fear of fat. I'm going to spend some time dealing with the fat issue, because it's so tied in with taste.

Fear of fat

You can't successfully tailor your tastes if you're afraid of fat. But if you are, it's no wonder. The 1980s and 1990s were fat-phobic decades—that's when it seems like every imaginable kind of food had a "fat-free" version. Fortunately, the scientific community and the media have increasingly recognized the health-promoting character of the Mediterranean diet—which features 40 percent of its calories as fat! And the beneficial effects of Omega-3 fatty acids (found in some fish, such as salmon) are becoming more widely known as well. With these developments, the excessive fear of dietary fat may be slightly abating.

However, decades of fat-phobia are hard to shake and, for many, counting fat grams and steering clear of fat is second nature. But take note: the fixation on fat grams is simply a repackaging of the same old calorie-counting diet message, this time substituting fat grams for calories. The focus is still on numbers rather than satiety and enjoyment of taste and texture.

To overcome this fear of fat, look around you and begin to critically evaluate the fat-obsessed language that people are using. Listen to the talk in the lunch room, pay attention to the commercials on television. The diet industry isn't talking about healthier eating when they push their "fat-free" products—they're just trying to fool us by putting a health spin ("low fat is healthier") on the old diet message.

What they're doing is transferring people's fear of body fat into a fear of *eating* too much fat. Yet, rigidly restricting your dietary fat, or replacing an obsession with body fat with counting fat grams, actually adds to your health problems by putting you back on the dieting track. So now's the time to ask yourself if you're substituting the fat trap for diet thinking. Take a look at how you feel about fat in the food you eat. The following focus questions will help you discover whether or not you, too, have been caught up in the fat trap:

- Am I counting the number of grams of fat in the food I eat?
- Do I base decisions about what to eat on the amount of fat in the food?
- Am I attempting to cut out all fat from my diet?
- Am I afraid of fat on my body and fat in food?
- Am I buying into society's view that avoiding fat is normal and healthy?
- Does my conversation revolve around food, fat, and fiber?
- Is this way of thinking causing me to obsess about numbers, calories, or fat grams or make me feel bad about myself?
- Am I restricting my fat intake to the point that it's inducing hunger, cravings, and feelings of deprivation?
- Do I binge on high-fat foods when I get the chance?
- Do I deny that I need to eat some fat for my physical health and enjoyment of food?

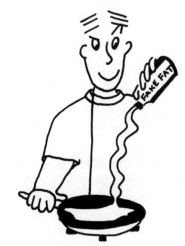

If you have answered yes to one or more of the questions, your answers have indicated that you've fallen into the fat trap. To set yourself free, it's time for a "fat reality check."

Is your diet too low in fat?

Part of the philosophy of listening to your body and tuning in to taste and texture involves making gradual changes, one step at a time. If you are getting cravings for foods high in fat, it may be a sign that you are not eating frequently enough or that you are restricting your fat intake too much. You will gradually acquire a taste for new foods that are lower in fat content. Remember, the new way of eating is for life! As you acquire your new tastes you want to avoid making yourself feel deprived— otherwise, your efforts to change your food habits won't last.

You are listening to your body and are eating an adequate amount of fat if:

- You are tuning into the texture, taste, and satiety value of the meal.
- You are enjoying the energizing feeling of balanced meals. Higher-fat meals make your mind and your body sluggish by slowing circulation and reducing the oxygen-carrying capacity of the red blood cells. However, meals too low in fat will leave you feeling hungry and thinking about food.
- You are accommodating your present taste preferences by making slight, gradual changes in your eating pattern.
- When you get hit with cravings, you're able to readjust the way you eat: making meals more regular and switching to more satisfying foods.
- You are paying attention to the experience of eating and allowing yourself to taste, savor, and enjoy your meals and snacks.

If, on the other hand, you answered no to some of these statements, it's time to reassess whether your diet is too low in fat. If so, you'll want to try to find a more normal and natural way of eating. A low-fat way of eating isn't for everyone all the time.

Enjoying the taste of health

I can't stress it enough: you need to learn to tune in to what your taste buds are telling you. But that doesn't mean you can't change the tastes you like. Here's a guide that can assist you to tune into changes while you're tailoring your tastes. Use the "New Experience" column to find ways to celebrate your positive reactions to leaner, less processed, more healthful foods.

Old Ways	New Experience
Appearance	
Grease floats on top of sauces, salads, soups. Vegetables look washed out. Beverages are thick (such as milkshakes). Grease leaves mark on napkin.	Food is refreshing, clean-looking. Sauces, dressings, garnishes all provide colorful accent without overwhelming the food. Brighter colors, more pronounced textures.
Taste	
Subtle flavors not noticeable. Flavors masked by fatty or sweet tastes. Sauces, dressings, and garnishes overwhelm food. Needs more salt or sugar to bring out flavors masked by fat.	Natural flavor can be tasted. Less salt and seasonings needed. Taste is subtle and builds gradually—the more you taste, the better it gets. Sauces, dressings, and garnishes enhance flavor without overwhelming.
Texture	
Mushy, gooey, soft, dense, greasy	Crunchy, crisp, chewy, clean
Mouth feel	
Coats mouth, greasy. Beverages leave mouth dry, coated with the fullness of the beverage.	Varies in texture and consistency. Beverages feel refreshing, go down easily.
Body response	
Feel heavy as the food goes down. Feel tired, bloated when finished with meal. Beverages leave you feeling still thirsty.	Refreshing, satisfying feeling as the food goes down. Not over-filling. Energizing. Beverages quench your thirst.

Taste Fundamental #3: Be Willing To Experiment

Whether it's a new pattern of eating, new foods, or new combinations of foods, it's important that you stay open to trying. And if something doesn't work this time, don't give up. Instead, try it a different way next time.

Now, that may sound difficult—especially if you're cooking for your family as well as for yourself. In fact, if yours is like many other busy families, you may rarely even manage to get together for a good, old-fashioned family dinner. But that's one tradition that's worth reviving—at least a few nights a week—for both nutritional and emotional benefits. Here are some great suggestions from my friend Jill on how to experiment with new foods, new ways of presenting them, and a new dynamic that will make the family dinner a much-anticipated part of the day.

- *Eat before dinner.* Yes, you read that right. When everyone in the family has become over-hungry during the meal preparation time, owly and snarly interchanges are highly probable. Combat this pattern with light snacking before the meal.

- *Ensure variety.* Variety can be a true spice of life at the table, but the main cook in your family doesn't want to get burnt out providing all that variety. So, don't expend one cook's resources: share planning, share list-making, share shopping, share cooking, and share clean-up.

- *Use style.* "Tastefully served food tastes better," is a phrase learned from my maternal grandmother that I'm proud to repeat. Both my grandmothers would position a slice of tomato with care and always prepared food with grace and appreciation. They used attractive accessories like unusual serving dishes, napkin rings, interesting placemats, and special table decorations. Their joy and pleasure in these touches was evident; I never detected an attitude of duty or obligation.

- *Nurture the art of conversation.* Encourage storytelling and anecdotes, wish lists and reminiscences. Trying to stimulate discussion with a "What happened in school today?" often doesn't open doors, whereas a nostalgic "When I was in eighth grade . . . " often inspires a lively telling of how different it is today. Guide ramblers to get to the point. Adult topic selection and opinion exchange will transmit values to the kids more effectively and naturally than a lecture on the subject.

- *Protect the mealtime.* Busy routines make a family meal together a precious opportunity to reconnect and build relationships. Phone calls don't have to be taken during the dinner hour—and if you *must* pick up the phone you can at least politely tell your caller "We're just eating, and I'll call you back in 20 minutes." You can make the house rules; don't be controlled by a ringing phone.

- *Scrutinize table manners.* Explore the relevance of rules like "no elbows on the table"; invent and fine-tune standards to your lifestyle. Ensure that the basic social necessities like "chewing with your mouth closed" are firmly entrenched to demonstrate respect for others.

- *Invite company more frequently.* Casual, collaborative meals with friends and family inject excitement and build up hospitality skills for all.

- *Instill surprise.* Who defines a special occasion? The surprise of a special meal or dessert in the middle of a routine week will be delightedly received. Arrive home with take out food from time to time.

Bring your children into the experiment

Jill's approach to family eating is based on a cultivated preference for nourishing eating patterns. I believe that your children can learn to trust their own tastes and body needs. Here are some adaptable suggestions that will enable you to experiment at your own table.

- *Creative education.* Help your kids discover what food does in the body, and why we need different kinds, in different combinations. Here are two examples of how you can use experimentation to help your children figure out the answers:

  1. Your kids come home from school. They're hungry and want a snack. Over time they've experimented with different combinations of foods for their after-school treat and discover that cheese and some cookies will give them the sustained energy they need to get to suppertime a few hours later. So they take a little of each—not lots of just one.

  2. Your kids are clamoring for you to buy the latest trendy breakfast cereal—they're *sure* it'll be all they need to get them through to lunchtime. Let them try it—they'll quickly discover they need more. Then let them try the cereal as a bedtime snack—it will probably be a better fit eaten this way, because at that point in the day they won't need sustained energy to fuel activity.

The point of these examples is that you want to be flexible about allowing your children to develop their sense of taste. Denying a taste experience because "it isn't good for you" or because it's not conventional is a form of the diet mentality.

Jill Says:

One evening my daughter was studiously ignoring her mixed vegetables, until she realized that if she claimed to be full now, she'd probably have to skip dessert—strawberry Jell-O with fresh strawberries. Looking me right in the eye, she dramatically put two fingers to her mouth and announced that she was turning off her taste buds to eat her vegetables. I was amused—and caught. After all, I knew there was just as much goodness in the dessert's strawberries as there was in the veggie portion she wanted to skip. I knew it, and so did she. She left the mixed vegetables on the side of her plate and had a large serving of dessert—and she even skipped the topping! I guess that some lessons have to be learned—and relearned!

- *Reasonable tasting expectations.* How do you or should you accept a child's claim that "I just don't like it"? And does one tiny spoonful qualify as a taste? The universal frustration of these familiar table maneuvers could sabotage your most patient intentions. Be a firm and imaginative guide as you suggest that the food is prepared slightly differently this time or "you've grown up a lot more now, you may be ready for a new taste."

- *An attitude and environment for experimentation.* "If that's all you want to eat, you'll likely be hungry very soon." Use this inevitability to demonstrate new food combinations. And be flexible; kids may prefer the chilled chicken from the fridge to the hot dish at the table. Try being more flexible in eating arrangements: If your child doesn't like the supper tonight, how about letting her help herself to yesterday's leftovers? It's certainly better than watching her pick at the food on her plate and then wind up snacking on junk food later on.

- *Allow your children to get hungry so they know what it feels like.* A regular eating pattern may not allow natural hunger to develop. Feed real hunger with different kinds of foods, and guide your children in the observation of how they feel after eating different combinations. This approach can be difficult, however, because it calls upon you to detach your sense of personal self-worth from the cooking process. In other words, you recognize that if the kids don't like the food, it does not reflect on your food preparation abilities or parental abilities.

- *Avoid the Good Food–Bad Food Trap.* Eating your vegetables doesn't make you a good person and eating dessert doesn't make you bad. The vegetables are not "good" foods and dessert is not a "bad" food. Be careful that you don't fall into this trap—and that you don't teach your children to fall into it either.

Taste Fundamental #4: Culinary Tricks of the Trade

Contrary to popular belief, fat belongs in your kitchen. It accents flavor, salads, and is essential to some cooking methods. But too much fat can coat your mouth with a heavy, creamy feel that hides the flavor and texture of the food. Here's how to find a happy medium:

- *Low-fat frying.* Cut the fat off meat before cooking. Brown meat quickly on both sides in butter, margarine, or oil to crisp and lock in flavor. Add fat-free broth for moisture, putting a lid on the pan to retain it. Gradually reduce the amount of fat in the pan until you've become accustomed to using a light spray of cooking oil.

- *Steaming or microwaving vegetables.* Boiling vegetables boils out the flavor and texture as well as nutrients into the water. Experiment with alternate methods, such as steaming and microwaving, to lock in the flavor and texture so that heavy sauces are not required to put flavor back. You may actually start to enjoy the natural taste of vegetables.

- *Use less oil.* Over time you can reduce the amount of oil in most recipes until it's about half what's recommended in the original recipe.

- *Use herbs and spices as accents.* Get creative about using those little jars in your spice rack. You'll find that you'll need less salt, sugar, or fat to flavor your foods, and you'll bring a new taste experience to your household.

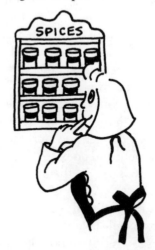

- *Change your approach to sandwich salads.* Tuna, ham, and egg salads in sandwiches are easily changed to tasty, lower-fat versions. For example, start with water-packed varieties for tuna or salmon salad instead of the variety that's packed in oil; or use broth-based chicken salad. If you're so inclined, you can gradually substitute the full-fat mayo with the lower-fat version, cutting back on the amount of dressing you use as your newly acquired tastes make it more appealing. And if you truly don't like lower-fat mayo, try reducing the amount of the real thing so that you moisten, rather than drench, your sandwich, or try substituting lower-fat salad dressing to moisten the salad.

Tailoring Your Tastes—In Action! *by Heather Wiebe Hildebrand*

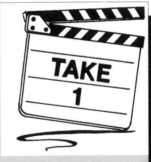

My husband Bernie grew up in a family where rich cream gravies were a wonderful part of several favorite ethnic dishes. Five years ago, when we started to incorporate gradual changes into our eating patterns, we decided to tackle the gravy that went with these foods. The gravy was originally made with cream, onions, butter, salt, and pepper. Our first gradual change was to move to half cream and half whole milk . . . we left everything else the same. The gravy was still delicious. We made it like that for four months before we moved to the next change.

The next step was to use one-quarter cream and three-quarters whole milk. The gravy wasn't quite as thick as we were used to, so we added a little cornstarch mixed with milk to make a paste to get the desired thickness. We kept this version for four to six months before we moved on. Eventually (after about two or three years of gradual change) we got to the point where we used evaporated skim milk and a little more seasoning, such as pepper and onions. We combine cornstarch with milk to thicken, and we still love the creamy gravy.

This past Christmas when we went to my husband's home his mother made us a traditional food—served with the traditional cream gravy. My husband took one bite and looked right at me. He smiled, nudged me, and said, "Heather, this is too rich, I'm not sure I can eat this." In a gentle way he explained to his mom that he would need a new plateful of the food without gravy on top. Then he used just a little gravy thinned with milk on the side to dip into for a little flavor. We were both pleased to see how our tastes had changed. We no longer even enjoyed the heavy mouth and body feel of the creamy gravy. We were eating lower-fat foods because we *preferred* them!

So how can you really get started with the *Tailoring Your Tastes* ideas? Watch it —many people fall into the "diet thinking" trap. They think that if a lower fat version of a recipe is good then the *lowest* fat version will be even better, no matter what their taste preferences might be. But jumping into the lowest fat version almost guarantees that the recipe will be abandoned, because the flavor isn't enjoyable.

Your best key is to look at your cupboard when you're not on a diet or trying to "eat healthy." Start with a variation that reflects the ingredients in your cupboard for the food you like to eat. Imagine you are like Jane in the following example.

If Jane is on a diet, she usually has ingredients in her cupboard that are low in fat, low in sugar, and high in fiber, even though she doesn't really enjoy these foods. They reflect the diet she is on, not her normal taste preferences. If she uses her cupboard to determine how to start tailoring her tastes, she would probably go right to the lowest fat options. This would set her up for failure, because she'll be preparing foods she doesn't really enjoy and probably won't stick to over the long term. It is important for Jane to think about the ingredients, the foods, and the flavors that she enjoys when she is eating normally and isn't dieting and use these for her parameters. In this way, Jane will have the opportunity to make small changes in the way she eats and cooks and may eventually enjoy the foods she once reserved only for diets (the ones she used to hate).

Recipe Concepts

In our book, *Tailoring Your Tastes*, my co-author Heather and I developed 53 detailed, kitchen-tested recipes that you can make exactly according to the directions. Now I'm going to share with you a recipe—plus variations—that illustrates some of the techniques you can use to healthfully make over any of your own favorite recipes. When you discover how one change might affect cooking time or behavior of the other ingredients in the recipe, you have absorbed the concept and can put it to use again.

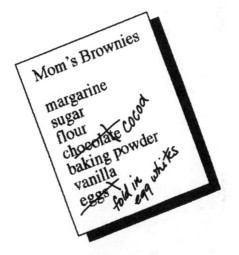

The recipe makeover

Step 1: Keep changes simple and gradual.

Step 2: Look at the recipe and the ingredients. Write down what areas in this recipe could use alterations to move them toward healthier eating. For instance, look at the recipe's fat, sweetener, salt, and fiber content and cooking process. Remember not every recipe will need changing in every area, and not every recipe needs to be changed.

Step 3: Once you have determined the areas that you would like to make changes, pick just two—say, changes in salt and fat content—then . . . GO FOR IT! Make small changes to these areas and remember to jot them down so you don't forget what you did.

Step 4: Try out the altered recipe and see what happens. Always make notes on how things turned out: how it tastes, how the texture, flavor, or aroma changed, and so on. If you didn't like the new version, make less of a change next time. If you did, stick with it for a few weeks or months before you go for the next change.

Step 5: Enjoy the process.

Always remember that there is no absolute right or wrong way to do this. The important thing is to make only about 2 (max: 3) changes per variation. Keep in mind that not every recipe needs to be changed in every area—and some of your traditional recipes won't need to be changed at all. But by all means be open to experiment with ideas and products, and avoid big jumps—they never seem to last, and your family won't appreciate them, anyway! Instead, once you've found a change you like, stick with it for awhile before you try to alter the recipe again.

Now, let's put all these principles into action! Here's a great muffin recipe from *Tailoring Your Tastes*. I'm including several variations—changes you can incorporate in the recipe gradually. Note how simple changes in ingredients and their proportions can have a substantial impact on the healthfulness of the recipe.

Sunshine muffins

Variations 1 yields 14 very large muffins or 20 to 24 smaller muffins; Variations 2 and 3 yield 12 to 15 large or 20 small muffins; variation 4 yields about 15 medium muffins.

These muffins are a delightful combination of flavors and textures. The ingredients make a moist, heavier muffin that is delicious. They are satisfying for lunch box or snacks. (Metric equivalents of measurements appear in parentheses in the recipe.)

Original	Variation 1	Variation 2	Variation 3
2 cups (500 ml) all purpose flour	2 cups (500 ml) all purpose flour	1-1/2 cups (375 ml) all purpose flour mixed with 1/3 cup (75 ml) whole wheat flour	1 cup (250 ml) all purpose flour, 2/3 cup (150 ml) whole wheat flour

1-1/4 cups (300 ml) sugar	1 cup (250 ml) sugar	2/3 cup (150 ml) sugar	1/4 cup (50 ml) sugar
2 tbsp (30 ml) baking powder	2 tbsp (30 ml) baking powder	2 tbsp (30 ml) baking powder	2 tbsp (30 ml) baking powder
2 tsp (10 ml) cinnamon	2 tsp (10 ml) cinnamon	2-1/2 tsp (12 ml) cinnamon	2-1/2 tsp (12 ml) cinnamon
1/2 tsp (2 ml) salt	Omit salt	1/4 tsp (6 ml) nutmeg	1/4 tsp (6 ml) nutmeg
2 cups (500 ml) shredded carrots	2 cups (500 ml) shredded carrots	2 cups (500 ml) shredded carrots	2 cups (500 ml) shredded carrots
1/2 cup (125 ml) raisins	1/2 cup (125 ml) raisins	1/2 cup (125 ml) raisins	1/3 cup (75 ml) raisins that have been soaked for 20 minutes
1/2 cup (125 ml) pecans or almond chunks	1/2 cup (125 ml) pecans or almond chunks	1/2 cup (125 ml) pecans or almond chunks	1/4 cup (50 ml) pecans or almond chunks, briefly toasted (less than 5 minutes) on metal sheet in 400[deg]F (200[deg]C oven) before adding to mixture
1/2 cup (125 ml) sweetened coconut	1/2 cup (125 ml) sweetened coconut	1/2 cup (125 ml) unsweetened coconut	1/4 (50 ml) cup unsweetened coconut, briefly toasted (less than 5 minutes) on metal sheet in 400[deg]F (200[deg]C oven) before adding to mixture
1 apple, peeled and grated	1 crisp apple, grated (leave peel on)	1 crisp apple, grated (leave peel on)	1 crisp apple, grated (leave peel on)

3 eggs	3 eggs	2 eggs	2 eggs
1 cup (250 ml) oil	2/3 cup (150 ml) oil	1/2 cup (125 ml) oil, 1/4 cup (50 ml) plain skim or 1% yogurt	1/4 cup (50 ml) oil, 3/4 cup (175 ml) plain skim or 1% yogurt
2 tsp (10 ml) almond or vanilla extract	2 tsp (10 ml) almond or vanilla extract	2 tsp (10 ml) almond or vanilla extract	2 tsp (10 ml) almond or vanilla extract

Mix flour, sugar, baking powder, cinnamon, and salt together in large bowl. Add carrots, raisins, nuts, coconut, and apple to the same bowl. Stir ingredients together. Beat eggs, oil, and extract in a separate bowl. Add liquid mixture to the dry ingredients and stir just enough to moisten. Place muffin mixture into muffin cups with paper liners, or spray muffin tins with a nonstick cooking spray. Fill each cup level to the top of the muffin tin. Bake at 350[deg]F. (180[deg]C) for about 20 to 25 minutes, or until a toothpick comes out clean.

NOTES:

Original Recipe: You may choose to omit either the raisins, the coconut, or the nuts. However, you'll end up with a change in flavor and texture, and there's be a decrease in yield.

Variation 1: There is no apparent change in flavor or texture in this version. The carrots and apple keep the muffins moist even though you use less oil and sugar. To make 20 to 24 smaller muffins, use smaller muffin cups rather than simply filling the larger ones to a lower level. Small muffins provide the same flavor, texture, and taste, and are the perfect size for a satisfying snack. When you include the apple peel, you add color, texture, and fiber, but note that the apples should be crisp if you plan on using the peel.

Variation 2: This variation yields fewer muffins because it uses less liquid and smaller amounts of other ingredients. There is, however, little change in the flavor of this version. Sweetness is maintained—even enhanced, by the sweet spices—cinnamon and nutmeg—and by the natural sweetness of the apples and carrots. In addition, cinnamon adds an appealing aroma during baking and afterwards. Unsweetened coconut gives tropical flavor and texture without adding extra sugar. Replacing all purpose flour with whole wheat increases fiber content, while decreasing the amount of egg in the recipe cuts back on fat and moisture content. The moisture of the muffins is maintained, however, by the apples, carrots, and yogurt used in the recipe.

Variation 3: These muffins have a bread-like texture—they're still moist, but a little more crumbly. Soaking the raisins makes them plump and juicy, so you need less of them to get the chewy texture and sweet flavor. Toasting the nuts and coconut intensifies their flavors, so you need less to get the same effect. The roasted taste and crunchiness in the muffins gives them wonderful texture.

Now, let's see how much difference these variations make in the nutritional value of the original recipe.

Nutrition Improvements	Variation 1	Variation 2	Variation 3
Salt	▼	▼	▼
Fat	▼	▼▼	▼▼▼
Sugar	▼	▼▼	▼▼▼
Fiber	▲	▲▲	▲▲▲

Here are a couple of general principles of recipe make-overs that you can take from the muffin recipe to use in lots of others:

- Plain yogurt can be used to replace moisture lost by decreasing the fat content when baking muffins and cakes.

- Nuts, coconut, and raisins are great additions to accent both flavor *and* texture. You can decrease their amounts and still get the satisfying crunch, chew, and flavor if you toast or soak them before using them in a recipe.

Of course, changing your recipes may mean changing the way you handle the results. For example, muffins made with decreased fat and sugar content don't stay fresh as long. But that's no problem—freezing them in an airtight container will help to preserve moisture and flavor. Then simply remove them from the freezer and thaw them in the microwave just before serving.

And while we're on the subject of recipe make-overs, remember, we're trying to make the food we eat *healthier*. We are *not* trying to ban any foods entirely. That's why, although many people are concerned about the cholesterol in egg yolks, you'll still see eggs used in the muffin recipe. The amount of egg per muffin is so insignificant that decreasing the eggs used in this recipe is not necessary.

Similarly, the recipe reduces but does not entirely eliminate sugar. A certain amount of sugar is necessary for both the texture and the taste of the muffins. As you begin to enjoy foods that are lower in sugar, however, you will discover that you like their more bread-like consistency, and you'll no longer expect a strongly sugary taste.

Taking It Deeper

- **On: Enjoyable Eating**

  1. Pick one of your favorite foods and eat it very slowly, enjoying every mouthful. Make a mental note of the taste and texture and how you feel. What did you discover about your favorite food? Do you still find it as enjoyable as you did before you ate it? Are you satisfied, or do you still want more?

  2. Make a list of some new, healthy foods you'd like to try—you can include family suggestions on this one, too—then add one or two every few days over the next few weeks. Keep track of the ones you like.

- **On: Taste Fundamental #1: Take Your Time**

  1. Contrast the Big Jump to the Smooth Slide. How does the Big Jump approach feed into a "healthy at all costs" mindset?

  2. Have you ever imposed your own version of the Big Jump on your family's eating habits? If so, share your humorous experiences.

- **On: Taste Fundamental #2: Respect Your Tastes**

  1. Referring back to your responses on the Fat Trap quiz, discuss your "yes" responses and what they may mean about your real feelings about fats in your food.

  2. Start a collection of eating articles from current magazines and analyze them to see if they are simply repackaging the diet message into counting grams of fat, counting fiber grams, or points. If you're unsatisfied with the level of coverage given to the non-diet

approach, write a letter to the editor—if we stand together, changes *can* occur. The message of a real alternative will be delivered.

3. Are you listening to your body and eating an adequate amount of fat? If not, reassess your eating patterns to see where you can make gradual changes to include more appropriate amounts of fats.

4. Discuss ways in which you can improve your own taste awareness and enlist it in your efforts to tailor your tastes. Consider a variety of factors: presentation, taste, mouth-feel, texture, and your body's response to different foods.

- **On: Taste Fundamental #3: Be Willing to Experiment**

1. Over the coming week, experiment with ways revitalizing the traditional family dinner. Incorporate some of Jill's suggestions if they seem appropriate, and consider other possibilities, such as using special serving dishes, decorations, or other "special occasion" items at your everyday meals.

2. Examine the way you impart a healthy-eating message to your children. How might you include them in the spirit of experimentation?

- **On: Taste Fundamental #4: Culinary Tricks of the Trade**

1. Discuss some cooking techniques that you can use to improve the health-value of your meals without sacrificing taste or texture. Can you suggest some that haven't been included in this section?

- **On: Tailoring Your Tastes, In Action**

1. Do you have any stories of applying gradual changes and then all of a sudden realizing that you actually "prefer" the healthier version, the way Heather and Bernie did? Discuss your own discoveries, and the scenarios that have created your change in taste.

2. If your tastes are not changing, examine the pace at which you are making your adjustments. Discuss what you might do to smooth your transition, so that the changes—when they do come—will be permanent.

- **On: Recipe Concepts**

  1. Try the muffin recipe makeover—remembering to take it gradually and get used to a new variation before moving on to the next one.

  2. Once you've gotten the hang of substitutions, take a favorite recipe of your own and explore variations that will let you gradually improve its healthfulness. Put these insights into action in your own kitchen.

Next Stop:
Buddy Support

13

What's a Buddy?
How Buddying Works
Up Close with the Buddy System
Relapses and Rebounds
Lessons from Penny and Kerri
Winding Up, Winding Down

Empowered by what you've read here, you may already feel confident that you can jump off the diet rollercoaster for good. And, hopefully, you can. But in the upcoming weeks, months, and years, a little extra support will make your commitment to a lifestyle without diets a whole lot easier. One of the most valuable means of support that I've discovered is mentoring, or the "buddy" system.

What's a Buddy?

A buddy is anyone who can help you stay committed to your choice of a nondiet lifestyle. Your buddy doesn't have to be someone you know—a buddy's principal credential is that he or she shares your commitment to a diet-free lifestyle. And the buddy system works both ways: Your buddy may serve as a mentor to you, or you may be the mentor. Most often, you'll find that you and your buddy will end up switching roles every so often, depending on who's most in need that day.

How Buddying Works

Communication is key to the buddy system. When you feel the urge to buy a fad diet book, you get in touch with your buddy to talk it out. If you're facing a brunch buffet and fear you'll overeat, work through those fears with your buddy. If you're tempted to stop exercising or to join up with a diet group, let your buddy know.

In other words, your buddy's there for you whenever you face a situation where you need support and encouragement in order to stick with a healthful, diet-free lifestyle. But while communication is the key aspect of buddying, you've got options as to how you get that communication done. You can communicate with a local buddy by phone or face-to-face, but these days there's a whole new way to get support, even if you don't have a buddy nearby: You can buddy up by *e-mail*. E-mail has proven to be a fantastic way of communicating—the medium lends itself to well-thought-out advice.

Up Close with the Buddy System

To show you just how valuable e-mail communication can be, two real-life HUGS buddies, dedicated to the idea of a diet-free lifestyle, have offered to share some of their e-mail exchanges. You've met one of them in earlier chapters: Penny, a HUGS graduate. Her correspondent is Kerri, who was just starting out in her quest for a healthy life without dieting when the buddy relationship first began.

After Kerri's initial posting to the HUGS message board, Penny responded with some helpful support. Over the course of the months that followed, some very wonderful discoveries took place. The exchange we'll be sampling here begins just before Thanksgiving, after Penny and Kerri had already exchanged three e-mail communications. In these early messages, Kerri was not yet dealing with nondiet lifestyle issues but focusing instead on her weight and her bad health (she has high blood pressure). We open with Penny's supportive, encouraging, pre-holiday message:

Dear Kerri,

I'm just packing and getting ready to go out of town for Thanksgiving and I thought of you. Yes, I really did, don't look so shocked (just teasing). Anyhow, the reason I'm writing is that I expected to hear from you over the weekend and I won't be back until Monday.

I used to dread the holidays but I'm actually looking forward to this one. I thought that having been in your shoes at one time, you might feel better if I gave you a little tool to work with this weekend. I'm not sure what kind of a celebration you have for Thanksgiving but if you're anything like I was, you get all self-conscious about what you'll eat and whether it's okay to have seconds and dessert. Well my friend, since you're on this new journey and you're doing so well I wanted to give you a bit of encouragement to get you through.

If you remember, HUGS is about empowering and embracing you. It's not about what you eat or when you eat or how much you eat; it's about how you feel. So, here's what you need to think about as you start the weekend. Thanksgiving is about giving thanks, it's not about the food. Forgive me if this is too religious for your tastes, but Thanksgiving was about giving thanks to God for the bountiful harvest. The harvest of food that would feed a family through a winter and possibly allow some to be sold for money. It's also about giving thanks for the plentiful trees for firewood.

For me, Thanksgiving is a time for giving thanks for the blessings I've received over the year. For the friends who have stuck with me through thick and thin, to the new friends and acquaintances that crossed my path, for the security of my husband's job so that I can continue to be home with my daughter and still be able to provide all the comforts we all need, for our good health, for our strength, for our new visions.

Yes, there is a big meal involved. I will be sitting down to a table with approximately 15 people. There will be a lot of food. Three women are contributing to this meal so you can just imagine the amount and the variety of food that will be there to eat, not to mention the dessert. How does that compare to what you're facing? Yes, I will probably have more to eat than I need. Yes, I'll probably have more to eat than I should. The difference for me now over other years is that I have learned to enjoy every single mouthful to its fullest. So here's what I'm suggesting you do for this meal and for every meal.

Sit down at the table and give thanks to yourself for being who you are, give thanks to yourself for doing positive things for the good of your health, give thanks to yourself for accepting who you are and then, if it suits you, thank God for inspiring you. Then as you dish out your plate take only those foods that you truly love the taste and texture of. Don't waste your time on things you don't enjoy (I always skip the Brussels sprouts). If you love mashed potatoes and gravy then take as much as you think you can ENJOY. The key here is to enjoy the meal. As you put a forkful in your mouth, savor each and every bit of it. Taste all the spices, the butter, the everything about every single morsel.

If you need to go back for seconds to fully experience the joy of the meal, then take seconds. The thing is, my friend, that by enjoying every single bite, you will eat slowly. In fact, you may find that something you thought you loved, you don't really care for all that much. You have to make a conscious effort to slow your meal down. But that doesn't mean you're being punished. It's not a trick. It's a treat.

If there is something new on the table, try it. I tried beets last year and found that while I don't really like them they did have a kind of interesting texture. Also, it was hard for me to learn that I didn't really have to clean my plate but you can clean it, that's okay too. The ONLY thing I want you to focus on during this weekend is the taste, texture, and enjoyment factor of everything you put in your mouth. Try not to let any guilt sneak in and stop you from enjoying your meals and desserts. If you're unsure about whether or not you can do this, try it at breakfast.

Really be passionate about your experience of fueling your body (eating). Listen to your body, and when you're full, stop. If you feel like you need to have more because it tastes so good, decide if you're going to have more or not and accept that decision. If the decision is to have more, then ENJOY it! If you don't enjoy it there is no point in having it. Remember too, it's okay to take some home! I love bringing leftovers home with me.

Write me soon and let me know how you made out. Let me know if you enjoyed this meal over any other. Promise yourself before you sit down at the table that you will not feel guilty and you will truly taste your food, paying attention to every bite. If there are a lot of emotional issues surrounding the table, which I know was a problem for me, then push them aside and make this meal about you and you alone. Don't use the food to push the feelings aside or down. Use the food as fuel to keep your energy up and enjoy the process of putting it into your body. Otherwise, what's the point in eating?

Happy Thanksgiving my new friend. I hope it truly is a happy one for you.

Penny

P.S. I hope I get a full report early next week!

The holiday came and went, but soon afterward Kerri responded to Penny's supportive Thanksgiving outreach. The first thing Penny noticed was how Kerri's attitude had turned around—this post-holiday e-mail showed that Kerri was beginning to see some light at the end of the nondiet tunnel.

Dear Penny,

I'm sorry I haven't written sooner. I've been so busy!! My Nana, cousin, and his wife and children were at my house for dinner last Monday night, Tuesday night we packed and tidied, and Wednesday we headed for Ottawa to visit Mike's dad and his Grandma: She received the Senior Citizen of the Year Award for Ontario. Kinda neat, eh? All of Mike's Dad's side of the family went out for dinner to help Grandma celebrate. (More eating!)

Kerri

*   *   *

Dear Kerri,

Congratulations for Mike's Grandma! That is very neat. All celebrations involve food. I think that it's been that way since the beginning of time. We're going to have to just learn to live with that. This is the reason that keeping in mind that food is a fuel can help. Eating is not a bad thing, your body needs that fuel.

Overeating is not a bad thing but when your car's gas tank is full do you keep filling? The key here is to put food in its proper perspective and treat it as a fuel and not as a lover. You say a lot of things later on that really show you already know this.

Penny

Dear Penny,

I read and re-read your letter and advice regarding Thanksgiving Dinner. I am still working on my first goal, which is to eat only until satisfied and not to overeat. I still get feelings of guilt if I overeat. That has to be the worst feeling. It's kind of like the angel on one shoulder and the devil on the other: "Yes, you deserve to have it" . . . "No, you should not even think of having it" . . . and usually the little devil wins. Do you know what I mean?

Kerri

*   *   *

Dear Kerri

Yes I know exactly what you mean. First of all, congratulate yourself for still working on the first goal and for recognizing that you haven't completely grasped how to listen to your own body cues! You're doing well just by knowing that you have to keep trying. Listening to body cues is hard but not impossible. The reason is, people like you and I have not been listening for a very long time.

I know for me learning what hunger felt like was the hardest thing to do. The second thing was recognizing the difference between thirst and hunger. Once I got that (and I do still struggle with it myself) I had to learn to properly respond. I found for me, eating breakfast was the hardest thing to do. But if I have a banana or apple or a juice before I have coffee, I feel the hunger, then I can eat my breakfast and know when I'm well fueled for the morning. If I get up and grab my coffee first (which I NEED to do) then I don't actually feel hungry and it's lunch before I realize I need fuel and then I'm in a bad cycle all day because I'm not well tuned into my body signals. It's a very hard thing to master and something I struggle with too.

Thirst is another. Especially at the end of the day. If I feel like munching when I know I shouldn't really be hungry, I try to drink water (when I'm really paying attention) but more often than not I'm reaching for diet pop (more caffeine and salt). I can honestly say that for me there is a connection between cravings/munchies and thirst. Lots of times a drink of water will kill a craving because it's my body asking for liquid. Sometimes it doesn't work, and that's when I know that I have an emotional thing happening. It's very hard to always be turned on and tuned in to what is going on with our body and mind, but ignoring those needs is what makes us do things to excess.

Penny

Dear Penny,

I tried to think of your words of wisdom and live by them. Savoring every bite and enjoying every mouthful. I don't think I ever really do that. I'm too busy trying to ensure everyone else has what they need and that everything is just perfect for everybody. I often put my needs after everyone else's. That causes emotional tension and then I do eat too much just to nurture myself and feel better.

Kerri

*   *   *

Dear Kerri

There is your answer Kerri. You do so much for everyone else that you ignore your own needs and then your emotional side kicks in and demands to be nurtured. It is a hard cycle to break out of. That's why HUGS is more about nurturing yourself first and fueling your body second. You just need to be more in touch with what your insides NEED, not what your heart desires.

Guilt is a killer. It's like a drug, you know. We learn guilt and shame as children and we use it like an addiction our whole life through. I already see that in my 4-year-old daughter. There is no shame nor guilt in overeating, Kerri. You need to work on believing that when you overeat, all you've done is missed a signal from your body. Either you missed the one that says "hey I'm full" or you've missed the one that says "hey, I need nurturing."

No matter why you overate, you didn't do it because you're weak or greedy. You did it simply because you weren't paying enough attention to yourself. You are working all the time on listening to body signals and if you happen to miss a few, fine. Give yourself a break and move on. You can't undo the overeating so let it go.

What happens to us, Kerri, is we overeat because we weren't listening to our body, then we feel guilt and shame, then we beat ourselves up for it so we feel bad so we try to feel better by eating something comforting so we feel guilt and shame and we beat ourselves up some more and we feel bad so . . . and on and on and on. Wouldn't it be better if we could say: "gosh, I ate more than I needed. I will try to pay better attention next time" and leave it at that? After all, the damage is already done. Why keep degrading and berating ourselves over it and making it worse? Learn to let that go and remove guilt and shame from your repertoire of feelings (very hard to do I know!)

Penny

Dear Penny,

I'm really trying to do things so that I will feel better. Things that don't involve eating but that are very pleasurable. Like having a bubble bath and talking to my girlfriends on the phone.

Kerri

*   *   *

Dear Kerri,

Good for you! You need to be pampered and nurtured. Don't forget that you need to fuel yourself too. Eating is a necessity but so are bubble baths.

Penny

*   *   *

Dear Penny,

I don't know if you're like this, but I always feel I have to be superwoman. I try to keep my house just so and do everything for my family and husband and dogs.

Kerri

*   *   *

Dear Kerri,

I used to feel that way. Then I realized that being superwoman actually meant knowing what my limitations were and knowing that I was a better person when I took the time to re-energize myself. Sometimes all I need is 10 minutes of sitting down to do cross-stitch and then I can usually see things more clearly. You know, Kerri, we don't need a lot of time. A few minutes makes a world of difference.

Penny

Dear Penny,

At the end of the day, there's not much energy or time left for me. Do you ever feel like that? That's when I find myself reaching for the chips. I'm truly not hungry, just emotionally drained.

Kerri

*   *   *

Dear Kerri,

I feel exactly like that and I try to deal with that every day. You hit the nail on the head there. Now just find your way of dealing with that. Like I said, for me 10 minutes when I feel out of control makes a huge difference. When I find that I'm reaching for the chips, I try (and often don't succeed) to just sit for a few minutes and let my head clear, or I get a drink of water and daydream, or I do a bit of stitching, or read a few paragraphs of a book I'm enjoying. I find 10 minutes is sometimes not enough, and sometimes I am just so emotionally charged or drained that I'm grabbing the bag.

Penny

*   *   *

Dear Penny,

Eating really is so psychological. It's surprising with so many weight-loss groups that the focus is not more towards the emotional end of it.

Kerri

*   *   *

Dear Kerri,

You have really hit the mark there! See, you know it, you just need to put it in practice.

Penny

Dear Penny,

I'm still not feeling very well. This blood pressure medication is really a downer. Side effects are very unpleasant. I hope I start to feel better soon. To be positive about things you really need to feel good.

Kerri

*   *   *

Dear Kerri,

Being on medication can make it tough. The only advice I can offer is to keep thinking, keep listening to your body, and keep doing what you're doing (nurturing yourself).

Penny

*   *   *

Dear Penny,

You know something else that is difficult to deal with, in my new way of thinking, is other people's views or comments. My Pappa is very conscious of my weight and does not hesitate to say, "Now Kerri, you don't need that. You won't lose weight eating that. Ah ah ah, that's enough!" That just drives me insane. And it's embarrassing. I've always been so careful to eat only what people think I should be having in public. Now, when I have something I want, but only one or two, people notice and think I've gone off my diet. I have actually. But I'm being careful in a different way. I'm extremely sensitive in every aspect of my life and those kind of comments just upset me. What do you think about that? Have you experienced this?

Kerri

*   *   *

Dear Kerri,

I do get a lot of pressure, from my mother-in-law mostly. I have learned to tune her out though. I used to fight and give my HUGS speech but I find now that I just let her talk and I let it all just go in one ear and out the other. My sister recently lost a lot of weight (again) but I'm sure she will find it again soon. I hadn't seen her for awhile and I was really terrified to see her. I didn't know how I'd deal with her comments. Then when she arrived she pointed out that I STILL looked like I was about 7 months pregnant (and yes that's the truth). I said to her very sweetly, "well thank you for pointing that out to me. I hadn't noticed it until you said." She had nothing to say after that. I don't know where I found those words, but they worked.

Kerri, we're never going to change public opinion completely. More and more people are jumping on the nondiet lifestyle bandwagon. More and more are realizing that dieting is harmful and is not the answer. It will take you a very long time and a lot of energy to make people understand that you are doing something positive for yourself. For right now, you have so much to concentrate on, you don't need to use what little energy you have dealing with people who will never understand anyway.

From my experience, what has worked is not letting myself get engaged in diet discussions. I have armed myself with self-righteous strength to know when enough is enough for ME. I don't worry about what others think even when they tell me what they think. When my mother-in-law did her "you know you don't need that" routine, I simply said, "you're right" and reached for it anyway. If she pressed on with a "then why are you having it?" then I replied, matter of fact, "because I want it." I know it's hard to do that to your Pappa and that it sounds disrespectful. But seriously, when dealing with those things, you need to (1) ignore them and (2) let them know somehow that you won't engage in that conversation.

Kerri, before much longer, you'll be doing things differently and those comments won't be made anyway. You will see. For now, just concentrate on you and your baby steps and those around you will follow your lead. It really does work like that.

I'm glad to hear such positive news from you Kerri. There really is a change in the way you present yourself and your ideas. Even if you don't see it yet, I do. Honest. Others around you will see it soon too. Keep up the great work. Keep in touch and let me know how things are going. You're helping me while I'm helping you and I do enjoy hearing from you too.

Penny

Relapses and Rebounds

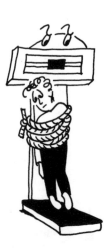

After a promising start, Kerri dropped out of communication with Penny for a short while, and tried handling her transformation to a diet-free lifestyle on her own. Sometimes we all have to take a step back, and sometimes this works to our long-term advantage—even if we see a short-term slide back into our old ways. For Kerri, a combination of family and health pressures made it increasingly difficult to "go it alone" in her diet-free lifestyle, and she suddenly popped back up in Penny's e-mail with a big surprise—she was going back to Weight Watchers!

Dear Penny,

Well hello there! I've thought of you often, but I just haven't been at the computer. I've been very busy with work and home life. Both have been crazy. I just looked at my last letter to you and it was at Thanksgiving. I'm not a very good pen pal. Ha!

I've been having a terrible time with my dieting or lifestyle change. Lots of stress and I just don't seem to react well to it. There has been sickness in my family and most upsetting of all, my beloved dog Bunny has lost her sight. She is completely blind and, after going to a dog ophthalmologist, she confirmed that her loss of sight was permanent and quite possibly due to systemic problems within her body. Our local vet is still checking into what has caused this problem. Her kidneys appear to be the problem. So far no cancer or heart disease has been found. Through it all, my sweet little dog has done so well. She was bumping into things and getting very scared, but she's starting to get used to her handicap. If only "mom" could! I cried all weekend and week worrying about her. Things are looking a little brighter though.

I don't know if I should tell you or not, but I rejoined Weight Watchers. I just felt that I needed a little boost to keep me going. I was very pleased to see I hadn't gained any weight. I've been doing fairly good until last week. The leader is very funny so it's quite enjoyable. I am still using my other tools but sometimes getting on the scales is a good scare tactic. I really, really want to lose this weight, once and for all. It is so unpleasant.

You would find this amusing possibly, but if I could just get to your size I'd be really pleased. Maybe some day!

Are you preparing for Christmas? I'm about half way there. I have lots to buy for though. I'm all decorated except for our tree. We'll get a real one the first weekend in December. I can hardly wait. I just love Christmas! Do you?

Well, I hope all is well with you and your family. Take care and I'll look forward to hearing from you when you get a chance. Bye for now.

Kerri

*   *   *

Dear Kerri,

I'm so sorry to hear about your dog. It's sad when someone we love is ill and we are unable to help. It's at those times that we turn to food for comfort, or in my case, to push the food down, down, down.

I'm glad you told me about Weight Watchers. I've often thought of it myself. The reason I haven't rejoined Weight Watchers is because I'm afraid to let myself slip back into that mode of thinking, where the scale controls me and I play the little food games to keep the scale as my friend. I'm not judging you for it, it's just never been a good experience for me. I understand they've changed the program quite a lot. I do hope it helps you. The HUGS tools will come in handy in helping to keep you focused on how you feel. Keep me posted on how you're doing.

I'm almost ready for Christmas. We're putting the tree up this weekend. I don't have many more to buy for. It will be good to get the preparations out of the way so I can enjoy the holiday. My daughter and I will be doing our cookie baking today actually. This year will be a true test of my success with HUGS. I have to tell you, for the first time in years and years, I'm not worried about the food.

Wishing you well! Happy Holidays!

Penny

Penny recognized that Kerri's e-mail was a call for help—and she did her best to provide support—but she realized that she didn't have all the answers. In fact, she identified with a lot of the troubles that Kerri was going through. Fearing that she might have let Kerri down, Penny, too, turned to a buddy for support and advice— me! Here's *our* e-mail exchange.

Dear Linda,

Here are the latest pieces between me and my e-mail friend. Please let me know if there's anything else I could add. I wasn't sure what to say to her. I was actually quite angry at first, but then I realized that I went through the same thing, only I didn't go back to Weight Watchers.

Penny

*   *   *

Dear Penny,

Kerri's return to Weight Watchers is not all that disappointing. She is simply going through the usual discovery process and needs some first-hand support. This does not mean that what you've said was not useful, nor does it mean that it will not stay in her mind. She did say that she will bring along the concepts, so maybe she just needs the group support that many of the diet programs offer.

When talking to some of my former clients, they tell me that they go to Weight Watchers for the support—not the diet or the concepts, just the support. So if there's no HUGS group in their community, this makes sense to me—and it's something that Weight Watchers *does* do well.

I would keep in contact with her. It doesn't sound like she wants you to stop mentoring her. Follow her through the process; see where it goes and what kind of conclusions she ends up having. Note the pattern, the journey. Kerri eventually might just realize that Weight Watchers' concepts are too diet-oriented through her own experience (often we do need to learn that way), and then she may come back to you with a different perspective. Hang in there.

Linda

Penny took my advice to heart—after all, her biggest concern was not to fail Kerri as a mentor. She kept the door open for Kerri to continue on as a buddy, providing a sympathetic "ear" while Kerri worked through her own problems and challenges. And, to Penny's great joy, Kerri *did* ultimately have a change of heart about Weight Watchers.

Dear Penny,

So sorry I've taken so long getting back to you. What a busy, busy time during the Christmas season. I hope you had a wonderful holiday season!

Mine was sad this year, as my Grandfather passed away on December 19, 1999. His absence at Christmas was very sad. He had always brought so much fun and laughter to our gatherings. I will miss him always. I was lucky in the sense that I had visited with him that night at the hospital and I was holding his hand as he died. I feel he knew he was not alone.

I wasn't working during the Christmas season, but it was not as enjoyable as it could have been with Pappa's passing and to add insult to injury, I got the flu on Christmas Day. I was entertaining my family as well, so the whole gang was here. Anyway, we got through it. I'm quite looking forward to 2000. I kind of had a crappy year in '99 with so many little issues arising and I feel positive this will be a better year.

Just to fill you in, I only lasted at Weight Watchers for 3 weeks before I got discouraged. I lost weight each week, but focusing weekly on how much I needed to lose only made my plight seem more hopeless than ever. Anyway, I am back to using my tools for better health from HUGS, and hopefully I will get my butt in gear and start exercising faithfully.

It truly is a long road, but one of my resolutions is to enjoy life now. I won't be waiting any longer until I lose weight to have fun or do things that I want. Just because I'm not slim doesn't mean I shouldn't enjoy social occasions, etc. What do you think?

I'm thinking about joining a low-fat cooking course, as I love to cook and that would be good to learn healthier methods that taste good. Also, I may join line dancing. I live in the country, so the weather is sometimes an issue, but so far it's been great . . . .

Thanks for all your help in the past and I look forward to chatting with you soon. Have a wonderful and healthy year!

Kerri

Dear Kerri,

I'm terribly sorry to hear of your Pappa's passing. I believe our loved ones never really stray too far from us. I hope that very soon you'll feel him close and whispering in your ear. I'm glad for both of you that you were with him as he left this earth.

Happy New Year! If you look through your computer screen right now, you should be able to see me dancing! I'm so happy to hear that you've grasped one of the hardest lessons HUGS teaches. Enjoy Life NOW! I'm not knocking Weight Watchers. Heaven knows I've thought about rejoining many times.

Like you though, the constant knowledge of how far away from goal I am always leaves me feeling defeated before I begin.

Did you get my mail about the closet cleaning? [Over the holidays, Penny had tackled the project of emptying her closet of all her old, too-small clothes. This project is described in Penny's Pearls in Chapter 7.] I can't stress enough what a good thing that is. I still cannot believe what a positive effect that has. I realized that having all those various sizes in the closet has the very same negative effect that the "goal weight" of diet thinking has on my mental state. Meanwhile, I am down a noticeable amount even over the holidays. People are commenting so there must be some change.

The best part of that closet-cleaning exercise, though, is the control I feel. I've still got 2 sealed boxes of chocolates in the house and only one that's open. It took me 2 weeks to enjoy a large Toblerone bar that, in the past, I would have devoured in a single sitting. That's a truly amazing milestone for me. The control is such a big deal for me, and something I've only just realized I had. This truly is a long road to travel. I've been at it now 3 years. Stick with it Kerri. In the long run you will be very pleased.

As for the rest of my life, well, I'm facing 2000 finally feeling like a whole person, and a grown up. It's about time, I think.

Lessons from Penny and Kerri

When you're trying to make a major lifestyle change, it's important to break it down into little, more manageable steps. But equally important is to feel that you're not trying to do it alone. Yet many of us lack a support system—or the people who *try* to support us—a spouse, our family or friends—slip into nagging, even though they have all the best intentions.

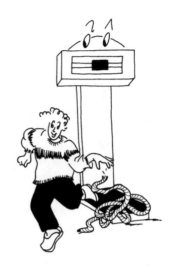

That's why buddying is so important. When the going gets tough, and we can't see instant changes, we all need somebody to remind us that our efforts are worthwhile. That's what Penny provided for Kerri—and what I provided for Penny, as well. Kerri knew that Penny would be there for her, and would understand what she was going through, because she knew Penny *had been through it too*!

Most important of all, she knew that, no matter what, Penny would keep the lines of communication open—even when Kerri went back to the Weight-Watchers program and its focus on dieting. And Penny's willingness to keep the door open—which all good buddies will do—made it possible for Kerri to find her way back to a diet-free lifestyle.

Winding Up, Winding Down

So—let's all jump off that diet rollercoaster! The principles you've learned in this book should give you the "parachute" you need to quit that up-and-down dieting lifestyle and come back to solid ground, where a healthier, happier, saner life waits for you. You, too, can find the confidence, self-esteem, and—yes!—freedom that a life without dieting has to offer!

Taking It Deeper

- **On: Buddy Mentoring**

    1. Discuss the benefits that the mentoring or buddy system provide. Examine the support resources available to you through your network of family and friends and in your community.

    2. If you have access to the Internet, go to www.hugs.com and explore the resources there. Don't worry—if you're not ready to post a message yet, you don't have to. But do feel free to look in at the

message board—once you see that there's a whole community of people sharing your goal, you just might feel bold enough to post a question or comment of your very own!

- **On: Penny and Kerri's E-mail Correspondence**

    1. Discuss Penny's guidance to Kerri in the pre-Thanksgiving e-mail. Identify specific points of guidance that you can identify with, and discuss how Penny's willingness to share her own experiences may help Kerri (and you) to cope with holiday food pressures.

    2. Penny stresses that guilt doesn't help when we overeat. Discuss this idea, and examine how you can apply it constructively in your own life.

    3. After the holiday, Kerri temporarily returned to the traditional, diet-oriented approach of Weight Watchers. What effect did her buddy relationship have on this decision? How might things have turned out differently if Kerri didn't have a buddy for support?

Appendix A

Meet the Ladies

Throughout this book you've had the chance to read the stories of a number of women who have adopted the diet-free lifestyle. Here's a little more information about these fine people.

Becky Chase, MS, RD: A former bulimic and compulsive eater, Becky knows first-hand that dieting encourages an obsession with weight. Today she is a HUGS facilitator and nutrition therapist in private practice in Colorado. She counsels individuals and groups specializing in nondiet approaches to meeting nutritional needs and maximizing health.

Heather Wiebe Hildebrand, RN, BSN: Heather, who shares her insights and experiences in "Take One" segments of this book, brings a distinctive perspective to diet-free living. As a person with diabetes, and as a health-care professional (she is a professional community nurse) she knows the importance of nutrition in maintaining optimal health. A HUGS facilitator, she is also my co-author of *Tailoring Your Tastes* (Tamos Books, 1995).

Carol Johnson: Carol is the author of the book, *Self Esteem Comes In All Sizes* (Doubleday, 1995). She graciously gave permission to use "Lose Weight and Call Me in the Morning," a chapter title from her book. Carol is also the founder of *Largely Positive, Inc.*, a Milwaukee-based organization dedicated to promoting health and self-esteem among larger people. For information on how to subscribe to the organization's quarterly newsletter, "On a Positive Note," send a self-addressed, stamped envelope to Largely Positive Inc., P.O. Box 170223, Glendale, WI 53217.

Christie Keating: Single parent, fitness instructor, former facilitator, and long-term HUGS member, Christie brings a thoughtful, poetic insight into the joy that comes from rejecting another ride on the diet rollercoaster. Her inspirational stories appear throughout this book, as she shares her "take" on everything from exercise to declaring "me" time for renewal and reflection.

Shelley McDonald: Three years after taking the leap off of the diet rollercoaster, Shelly remains enthusiastically committed to a lifestyle without diets. She proudly reports that she has succeeded in making activity a regular part of her life (she's taking up running!) and is realistic enough to forgive herself for the occasional relapse into the old diet mentality: "Sometimes I don't acknowledge my real needs, but now that's the exception, not the rule."

Heidi Mead: Our adventurous sailor (see Chapter Seven's essay, "Riding High and Free"), Heidi Mead is a long-term HUGS member and strong proponent of living life free from diets. Sounds like Paradise!

Kerri Miller: Kerri graciously gave us permission to excerpt her "buddy" communications with mentor Penny Muir (see Chapter 13) during her early exploration of the diet-free lifestyle. She's once again left Weight Watchers and is working at overcoming her old "diet thinking" so that she can fully enjoy the benefits of a truly diet-free lifestyle.

Penny Muir: A HUGS participant since 1997, Penny Muir (who gives us "Penny's Pearls" throughout the book, as well as excerpts from her buddying session with Kerri in Chapter 13) is a HUGS on-line mentor who's proud to share her strength and experience with others who seek to adopt a lifestyle that's free from dieting. Whether she's working out with her 3-year-old personal trainer (her daughter, see Chapter Nine) or gearing up for the annual International No-Diet Day, she puts her HUGS training into practice every day.

Wendyl Nissen: Wendyl has long been a committed advocate of the diet-free lifestyle. She is the former editor of *New Zealand Woman's Weekly*, a major women's publication that features articles on issues of particular interest to women.

Sandra Olafson: Sandra remains committed to "discovering the new stronger happier and healthier me" that living a diet-free lifestyle has brought her. She jumped off the diet rollercoaster when she turned 40 and since then has founded her own HUGS group to help spread the message of freedom from dieting to others.

Heather Todd: Heather is twenty-one and a student at the University of Manitoba, majoring in Occupational Therapy. Although she continues her seven-year struggle with an eating disorder, she is taking positive steps to overcome it through the diet-free lifestyle. She brings us all a message of hope: "I believe if we all learn to value ourselves for who we are, not what we look like, we will all be much happier people." She still journals.

Tanis Rempel: Another University of Manitoba student, Tanis is preparing for a career in Athletic Therapy. She is a strong voice countering the pressures of a diet-obsessed media. As she puts it: "The emotional and physical damage caused by [media] influence has encouraged me to step back and examine my own frame of mind. I had to stop allowing the unrealistic ideals to influence me, and start concentrating on living up to my own expectations." Her mom, Jan Rempel, adds these words: "Tanis has confidence in her ability and what she wanted to do, and society wasn't going to dictate what she became. She is adventuresome and not afraid to be her own person."

APPENDIX B

The Diet Mentality Quiz

Refer to Chapter 1, page 4 for scoring instructions.

The diet mentality quiz
Score: 1 = always; 2 = very often; 3 = often; 4 = sometimes; 5 = rarely; 6 = never

_____ I am unhappy with myself the way I am.

_____ I am preoccupied with a desire to be thinner.

_____ I weigh myself several times a week.

_____ I am more concerned with the number on the scale than my overall sense of well-being.

_____ I think about burning up calories when I exercise.

_____ I am out of tune with my body for natural signals of hunger and fullness.

_____ I eat for other reasons than physical hunger.

_____ I eat too quickly, not taking time to focus on my meal and taste, savor and enjoy my food.

_____ I fail to take time for activities for myself.

_____ I fluctuate between periods of sensible, nutritious eating and out-of-control eating.

_____ I give too much time and thought to food.

_____ I tend to skip meals, especially early in the day, so I can "save up" my food for one big feast.

_____ I engage in all-or-nothing thinking.

_____ I try to be all things to all people.

_____ I strive for perfection in my life.

_____ I criticize myself for not achieving my goals.

The diet mentality quiz

Score: 1 = always; 2 = very often; 3 = often; 4 = sometimes; 5 = rarely; 6 = never

_____   I am unhappy with myself the way I am.

_____   I am preoccupied with a desire to be thinner.

_____   I weigh myself several times a week.

_____   I am more concerned with the number on the scale than my overall sense of well-being.

_____   I think about burning up calories when I exercise.

_____   I am out of tune with my body for natural signals of hunger and fullness.

_____   I eat for other reasons than physical hunger.

_____   I eat too quickly, not taking time to focus on my meal and taste, savor and enjoy my food.

_____   I fail to take time for activities for myself.

_____   I fluctuate between periods of sensible, nutritious eating and out-of-control eating.

_____   I give too much time and thought to food.

_____   I tend to skip meals, especially early in the day, so I can "save up" my food for one big feast.

_____   I engage in all-or-nothing thinking.

_____   I try to be all things to all people.

_____   I strive for perfection in my life.

_____   I criticize myself for not achieving my goals.

INDEX

A

affirmations: 7, 22, 37

Afraid to Eat: Children and Teens in Weight Crisis: 23

all-or-nothing thinking: 4, 43, 73, 94–95

attitude: 3, 5, 7, 35, 44, 48, 122, 156

B

balance: 2, 23, 72–74, 146, 148, 173

Beauty Myth, The: 104

Berg, Francie: 23

Big Jump, the: 178–181

bingeing: 16, 18, 140

blood pressure: 20, 49, 54–55, 56, 116, 208

blood sugar:16, 49, 144, 164, 172

buddy: 2, 3, 35, 61, 120, 199–216

C

calories: 2–4, 14–16, 18, 23, 43, 51, 113, 145, 150, 161, 183

carbohydrates: 23, 129, 141–142, 146, 151, 160, 170, 177

Chatelaine: 159

chat room: 7, 76

children: 17, 23. 25, 27, 61–62, 133, 187–188

cholesterol: 49, 112, 113, 116

compulsive overeating: 20

confrontations: 22–23

cravings: 16, 28, 36, 141, 157, 160, 166, 172, 184, 185

Chase, Becky: 20

D

dehydration: 146, 148

depression: 18, 76

diabetes: 49, 54, 56

diet drinks: 150

diet industry: 162–163

diet mentality: 2, 3–5, 32, 35, 36, 41, 42, 44, 56, 114, 178, 187

diet rollercoaster: 2, 7, 14, 17, 63, 72, 140

diet talk: 32, 34, 35

doctors: 9, 48–58

E

eating disorders: 19, 21, 23, 84

Ecclesiastes: 60

electrolytic imbalance: 17

email: 7, 9, 200–215

energy: 18, 23, 26, 117, 122, 129, 141, 162, 165, 207

exercise: 2, 3, 18, 32, 49, 51–2, 55, 56, 101, 110–125, 126–138

F

fad diet: 14, 200

fat, fear of: 8, 14, 17, 182–183

fashion industry: 100, 103–104

fertility: 17

fiber: 8, 192, 195

fitness: 25

food record: 155, 163–173

freedom words: 34

G

glycogen: 15, 129

guilt: 2, 33, 35, 75, 166, 202, 205

H

heart disease: 49

heart muscle: 17

Hildebrand, Heather Wiebe: 8, 51, 94, 102, 132, 190

hormones: 16

HUGS: 6–7, 8–10, 22, 26, 33, 35, 51–53, 56, 60, 64–65, 72, 75, 82–83, 102, 176, 200–201, 205, 208, 211–214

hunger: 9, 16–19, 25, 36, 41, 43, 94, 129, 138–154, 156, 158–160, 164, 204

hypothalamus: 18

I

insomnia: 18

International No-Diet Day: 9, 52, 98, 99

irregular heartbeat: 17

J

Jenny Craig: 2

Johnson, Carol: 53, 54

journaling: 66, 82–84, 154–174

Journal of the American Medical Association: 112

K

Keating, Christie: 26, 52, 74, 96–97, 102, 135

L

Largely Positive: 55
Letterman, David: 19
low carb diets: 15, 141
low fat: 39, 149, 176

M

malnutrition: 20
McDonald, Shelley: 41, 122
Mead, Heidi 104–106
measure of success: 2, 3, 5, 8–10
media: 8, 100
medication: 208
Mendelson, Rena A.: 41
menopause: 162
menstruation: 17
metabolic rate: 18, 23, 112, 122
"me" time: 75
Muir, Penny: 8, 22, 56, 62, 76, 83, 90, 95, 96, 97, 121, 130, 143, 144
muscle loss: 15

N

New Zealand Woman's Weekly, 27
Nissen, Wendyl: 27

O

obesity: 9, 20, 54–55
Olafson, Sandra: 42, 159
overeating: 20, 61, 143

P

PAST technique: 77
Penny's Pearls: 8–11, 56–57, 62, 76, 90, 96, 97–99, 121–122, 130–131
personality: 18
PMS: 160–162, 171–172
pregnancy: 17
Priest, Ruth: 14
problem areas: 97
protein: 15, 24, 141–142, 150, 177, 179

R

Radiance Magazine: 14
recipe makeover: 191–192
rehydration: 129, 144, 147, 163

relapse: 5, 6, 210
Rempel, Tanis: 100–101

S

salt: 8, 148, 191, 195, 204
scales: 2, 4, 9, 23, 38, 44, 53, 210–11
self esteem: 16, 19, 20, 22, 28, 37–8, 43, 53, 60–61, 62–63, 79, 82, 88–109
set point: 18, 23
shortcuts: 79–80
single parents: 74
size discrimination: 94
Smooth Slide, the: 178–181
snacks: 37, 141, 143–146, 165, 180, 182
"So What" technique: 77
stages of change: 5,6
stress: 17, 70–87, 144, 210,
sugar: 8, 16, 49, 148, 192, 195, 196
Sunshine Muffins: 192–195
support: 2, 3, 7, 8, 60–69, 74–75, 93, 159, 199–216

T

Tailoring Your Tastes: 8, 176, 191, 192
Take One: 51–52, 94–95, 102–104, 132–133, 190–191
Take Two: 26–27, 52–53, 74–75, 97, 135–136
texture: 24, 202, 142–143, 177, 180–181, 184, 189, 202
thirst: 204, 138–154
Todd, Heather: 84
Top Ten: 19

V

vacation: 81–82
vitamins: 160, 173

W

water: 15, 146–152, 204
water weight: 15
Weigh-In Cheats: 19
weight regain: 14–15
Weight Watchers: 210–215
"Who's In Charge": 91
Wolfe, Naomi: 104
World Health Organization: 116

Y

You Count, Calories Don't: 9, 41, 63, 162–163, 172

BIBLIOGRAPHY

For Further Reading

Books

Berg, Frances M. *Children and Teens Afraid to Eat: Helping Youth in Today's Weight-Obsessed World*, Healthy Weight Network, 2001.

Berg, Frances M. *Women Afraid to Eat: Breaking Free in Today's Weight-Obsessed World*, Healthy Weight Network, 2000.

Jonas, Steven and Linda Konner. *Just the Weigh You Are: How to be Fit and Healthy, Whatever Your Size*, Chapters Publishing, 1997.

Johnson, Carol. *Self-Esteem Comes in All Sizes: How to Be Happy and Healthy at Your Natural Weight*, Doubleday, 1996.

Omichinski, Linda. *You Count, Calories Don't*, HUGS International Inc., 1999

Omichinski, Linda and Heather Wiebe Hildebrand. *Tailoring Your Tastes*, Tamos Books, 1995

Poulton, Terry. *No Fat Chicks: How Women Are Brainwashed to Hate Their Bodies and Spend Their Money*, Key Porter Books, 1996.

Publications

Radiance: The Magazine for Large Women. P.O. Box 30246, Oakland, CA, 94604

Websites

Healthy Weight Network: www.HealthyWeightNetwork.com

HUGS: www.hugs.com

Largely Positive, Inc.: www.largelypositive.com

Radiance Magazine: www.radiancemagazine.com

After the Diet: www.afterthediet.com

Help From HUGS

Starting your own HUGS support group

Making a major change in your life is always easier when you have friends to help you stay on track. That's why support groups are so important. But what if there are no support groups in your area? How about starting your own?

You, too, can become a certified HUGS support group leader. Here are some of the reasons why:

- Starting a support group helps you maintain and grow in your lifestyle without diets, providing regular reaffirmation of your decision to stay off the diet roller coaster.
- Leading a support group gives you a powerful opportunity to nurture your leadership skills through the HUGS Support Group Leaders Network.
- Linking your support group to HUGS lets you tap into the website's broad popularity when you're looking to advertise your group's activities and services.
- Joining the HUGS family provides you an opportunity to make money.

Starting the certification process is easy. Simply contact www.hugs.com, and HUGS International Inc. will provide you with an interactive resource package that will train you in the concepts that stand behind a diet free lifestyle. The training process takes about ten weeks. After you've completed the training, you're eligible for a one year license indicating you are able to deliver HUGS support groups in your area.

Log on to www.hugs.com for more details on the HUGS program and the certification process.

Products and Services HUGS International Inc.

Here's an array of products and services designed help you stick with the healthy living process. For items marked with an asterisk add $5.00 per item to cover shipping and handling.

You Count, Calories Don't, by Linda Omichinski, RD (HUGS International, 1999). Discover how to decide when and what to eat, set realistic goals about your physical size, and stop dieting and start living. U.S. $19.95/Can. $24.95

Tailoring Your Tastes, by Linda Omichinski, RD, and Heather Wiebe Hildebrand, RN (Tamos Books, 1995). An innovative cookbook that teaches you to follow a four-step transition to healthier eating—without sacrificing your enjoyment of food. U.S. $14.95/Can. $19.95

Staying Off the Diet Rollercoaster, by Linda Omichinski, RD (AdviceZone Books, Washington, D.C., 2000). U.S. $17.95/Can. $24.95

HUGS Affirmation Tapes, by Linda Omichinski, RD. Build self-esteem, increase diet-mentality awareness, use positive language, create a relaxed state of mind, be more assertive and more reflective. Set of 3 tapes. U.S. $33.95/Can. $41.95

Guided Journal: Keeping a Food/Hunger/Events Journal. Your own personal check-up for eating habits. A professional individual assessment of one week of your journal will show to what extent your lifestyle is in balance. Suggestions provided. U.S. $60.00/Can. $85.00

HUGS at Home program: A comprehensive resource package that will enable you to experience the next best thing to an actual HUGS class led by a licensed facilitator. Includes Guided Journaling U.S. $199.00/Can. $249.00

HUGS Club membership: Support group over the web to continue your diet-free life. Includes weekly encouraging e-mail from a group leader and access to the e-mail buddying system. Password protected. Annual membership U.S. $25/Can. $35

To learn more about any of these materials and any of our other programs, log on to www.hugs.com. You can order by fax, toll-free line, or by mail.

HUGS International Inc.
Box 102A RR#3
Portage la Prairie
Manitoba R1N 3A3
Canada

Phone order line (U.S. and Canada): 1-800-565-4847
Fax order line: 1-204-428-5072
Email orders: www.hugs.com

HUGS Order Forms

Please sent a copy of this form, with payment, to:

HUGS International, Inc.
Box 102A, RR#3
Portage la Prairie
Manitoba R1N 3A3
Canada
fax: (204) 428-5072

NAME _____

ADDRESS _____

CITY _____ STATE OR PROVINCE _____

COUNTRY _____ CODE _____

HOME PHONE _____ WORK PHONE _____

I would like to purchase the following:

☐ *You Count, Calories Don't.*   Qty:_____   Total:_____

☐ *Tailoring Your Tastes.*   Qty:_____   Total:_____

☐ *Staying Off the Diet Rollercoaster.*   Qty:_____   Total:_____

☐ *HUGS Affirmation Tape Set.*   Qty:_____   Total:_____

☐ *Guided Journal.*   Qty:_____   Total:_____

☐ HUGS at Home Program.   Qty:_____   Total:_____

☐ HUGS Club membership   Total:_____

Method of Payment:

Check: _____

Visa Card Number: _____

Mastercard Card Number: _____

If paying by credit card, please include expiration date: _____

Signature: _____

ABOUT THE AUTHOR

Robyn Ryle is an associate professor of sociology at Hanover College in Hanover, Indiana, where she has been teaching sociology of gender and other courses for 13 years. She went to Millsaps College in Jackson, Mississippi, for her undergraduate degree in sociology and English with a concentration in women's studies. She received her PhD in sociology from Indiana University. She is a member of the American Sociological Association and Sociologists for Women in Society and has served on the editorial board of the journal *Teaching Sociology*. She grew up in a small town in Northern Kentucky and now lives in another small town just down the Ohio River. When she's not teaching classes, she writes, gardens, plays the fiddle, and knits. She currently lives in a 170-year-old house in scenic Madison, Indiana, with her husband, stepdaughter, and two peculiar cats. You can find her on Twitter (@robynryle), on the Facebook page for *Questioning Gender* (https://www.facebook.com/questioninggender?ref=hl), or at her blog: you-think-too-much.com.